How We Think About Dementia

How We Think
About Dementia

Personhood, Rights, Ethics, the
Arts and What They Mean for Care

Julian C. Hughes

174.

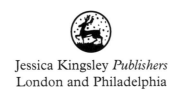

Jessica Kingsley *Publishers*
London and Philadelphia

First published in 2014
by Jessica Kingsley Publishers
73 Collier Street
London N1 9BE, UK
and
400 Market Street, Suite 400
Philadelphia, PA 19106, USA

www.jkp.com

Library of Congress Cataloging in Publication Data
Hughes, Julian C.
  How we think about dementia : personhood, rights, ethics, the arts and what they mean for care / Julian C. Hughes.
     pages cm
  Includes bibliographical references and index.
  ISBN 978-1-84905-477-5 (alk. paper)
  1. Dementia. 2. Dementia--Philosophy. 3. Dementia--Patients--Care. I. Title.
  RC521.H844 2014
  616.8'3--dc23
                                    2013050309

British Library Cataloguing in Publication Data
A CIP catalogue record for this book is available from the British Library

ISBN 978 1 84905 477 5
eISBN 978 0 85700 855 8

Printed and bound in Great Britain

To Sister Catherine Hughes SND
for being extraordinary in so many ways

Acknowledgements

I should like to thank: the Nuffield Council on Bioethics for permission to use material contained in Box 4.1, along with other quotes from *Dementia: Ethical Issues* (2009); Fondation Médéric Alzheimer for use of amended material in Chapter 9, which originally appeared in *Supporting and Caring for People with Dementia Throughout End of Life*, published in *Les Cahiers de la Fondation Médéric Alzheimer* in 2006 (pages 17–22); Solicitors for the Elderly, for use of amended material from 'Searching for Settled Practice', originally published in *Elderly Client Adviser*, 14, 1, pages 26–29 in 2008; SAGE publications for the use of Figure 11.1 and Box 11.1, taken from van der Steen *et al.* (2013); and Alzheimer's Australia for use of elements in Table 11.3, which originally appeared in an extended form in their Paper 35, 'Models of Dementia Care' which I authored in 2013 (Hughes 2013b).

Tatsumi Orimoto very generously made available to us a selection of pictures featuring him with his mother, from his *Art Mama* series, one of which we have used with his permission in Chapter 13. John Killick has kindly granted permission for us to use the poems or extracts of poems authored by him in Chapter 14.

I have expressed my sincere gratitude to Ashley McCormick in the Preface, but would like to acknowledge her permission to use 'no ifs, ands, or buts' in Figure 13.1.

I have tried to seek all appropriate permissions, but apologize for any oversights, which I would wish to rectify in any future editions of this book.

Contents

Abbreviations 9

Preface 10

Introduction 17

Part I Ageing

Chapter 1 Our Changing Expectations of Life:
What Do We Really Want? 26

Chapter 2 Research, Ageing and Dementia 35

Part II: Personhood

Chapter 3 Memory: Inner or Outer? 56

Chapter 4 I Am Still the Same Person 66

Chapter 5 The Body in Dementia 76

Part III Capacity and Incapacity

Chapter 6 'Capacity': What Is It and So What? 92

Chapter 7 Capacity Legislation in Practice:
Balancing the Personal and the *Polis* 109

Chapter 8 Incapacity and Mental Disorder 127

Part IV Palliative and Supportive Care

Chapter 9 Beyond Hypercognitivism   142

Chapter 10 Understanding the Language of Distress   151

Chapter 11 Ethics, Patterns, Causes and Pathways:
In Pursuit of Good Palliative Care   165

Chapter 12 Intentions and Best Interests:
Dying and Killing   186

Part V Arts

Chapter 13 The Art and Practice of Memory
and Forgetting   202
Julian C. Hughes and Ashley McCormick

Chapter 14 In Praise of 'Negative Capability':
Keats and Killick   219

Conclusion Care – Solitude and solidarity   226

REFERENCES   230

FURTHER READING   239

SUBJECT INDEX   240

AUTHOR INDEX   247

Abbreviations

§ signifies paragraph number in Wittgenstein citations

ADRTs Advance Decisions to Refuse Treatment

CPN Community Psychiatric Nurse

DoLS Deprivation of Liberty Safeguards

DSM-5 Diagnostic and Statistical Manual (5th Edition)

GDP Gross Domestic Product

GP General Practitioner

IMCA Independent Mental Capacity Advocate

LPA Lasting Power of Attorney

MCA Mental Capacity Act 2005

MCI Mild Cognitive Impairment

MHA Mental Health Act 1983

NHS National Health Service

PEG Percutaneous Endoscopic Gastrostomy

SEA situated embodied agent

VBP values-based practice

Preface

How we think is crucial. Many people reading this book will be involved – as family, as close friends or as professional carers of one sort or another – with people with dementia, and some may be living with a diagnosis of dementia. The difficulties that can arise in connection with dementia cannot be made light of, but nor should they be made more of than is necessary. These difficulties are often practical and, for understandable reasons, people will be looking for practical answers to the problems they face. In an earlier book published by Jessica Kingsley, Clive Baldwin and I argued that ordinary care involves an ethical component and that, in effect, many of the practical problems we face are also ethical in nature (Hughes and Baldwin 2006). The present book is not about practical problems. It is about how we think.

What I want to argue, however, is that how we think about dementia is crucial to how we react to it and, ultimately, to what we do about it. So this book is an unabashed attempt to clarify some of our thinking. I am inclined to feel that the fascination of dementia stems in part from the deep issues that it throws up about our standing as human beings in the world. This has two implications: first, some of our thinking about dementia needs to be about other things, such as about what it means to be a person, about human rights, about ethics and about art; second, given the profound nature of the issues which arise, and their breadth, I am sure that I shall not do the subject justice. We need more thinking about dementia by better minds than mine; and I apologize in advance for the deficiencies in my account.

In a sense, then, this book continues the theme from the earlier book with Clive Baldwin, but here I wish to dig a little deeper and wider. I am not going to be focusing on particular ethical dilemmas in detail. My intention is to look at the background to those dilemmas. Sometimes this will involve conceptual clarification, but sometimes it will involve setting out other features of our lives that influence our intuitions and judgements. My hope is that this will be seen as relevant to things that we actually do. Thinking right engenders doing right. At least, we need to be thoughtful in our dealings with dementia.

You might think I meant to say we should be thoughtful in our dealings with *people* with dementia. Of course we should. But part of what I am interested in is the concept of dementia itself and how this, in turn, affects our dealings with actual people. This book also represents a development of some of the ideas in my earlier book *Thinking Through Dementia* (Hughes 2011a). It is a development in the sense that I shall be adding some colour to the discussion in the earlier work.

One of my aims in *Thinking Through Dementia* was to raise questions about the concept of 'dementia' itself. In fact, I rejected it as a useful term and instead suggested that, if we need a heading in our systems of classification for the group of conditions usually referred to as 'dementia', we should talk of 'acquired diffuse neurocognitive dysfunction'. I shall not rehearse my reasons for thinking this would be better descriptive terminology. It is only better, of course, if you are interested in systems of classification (and you would still need to give some sort of pathological specification by talking of Alzheimer's type, or vascular pathology, or Lewy bodies, or whatever). If you think my suggestion is bonkers, then you have to keep in mind that subsequently the American *Diagnostic and Statistical Manual* (DSM) has appeared in its fifth edition (DSM-5), in which dementia is now referred to as 'major neurocognitive disorder'. I still prefer my terminology! This is in part because I prefer to think of things not working as well as they once did, rather than to hammer home the idea of 'disorder'. Part of the worry is to do with stigma and, for this reason, in the earlier book, I was disinclined to use the word 'dementia' at all. But in this book I shall stick to 'dementia' as if it were unproblematic, but this is only for pragmatic reasons: it's short and it's understood (although I am not sure how widely or fully, despite increasing publicity).

The book is based on a number of talks that I have given over the last few years. Only one or two of the chapters have been previously published (see Acknowledgements). There are two consequences. First, although some of the chapters are only loosely based upon the original talks, which I have updated and often extensively rewritten, nonetheless there are places where the content reflects the concerns at the time. So, for instance, some of the chapters about capacity were originally conceived before the Mental Capacity Act 2005 came into effect. I have chosen to leave some of the material much as it was, partly because I believe the issues are still relevant, but also because it sometimes seemed appropriate to record the concerns as they then appeared.

The second consequence is that I should thank the individuals or institutions which encouraged me to pursue the original work. This is, of course, a great pleasure. Chapter 1 first saw the light of day at a hugely enjoyable conference held in Cumberland Lodge in November 2010. I am grateful to everyone involved, but particularly to Professor Tom Kirkwood for inviting me and making this possible. The inspiration for Chapter 2 was originally also connected to Professor Kirkwood, because it came from a symposium about the goals of ageing research held in the Policy, Ethics and Life Sciences (PEALS) Research Institute in Newcastle University at the time of Professor Kirkwood's Reith lectures back in 2001. My good friend Dr Tom Shakespeare organized the symposium, the full proceedings of which can still be read on the PEALS website (Hughes 2001a). The chapter has, however, been completely rewritten, although the thoughts behind it were generated in that symposium. Chapter 3 is based on the 'Holding Memories' Workshop held at Newcastle University in September 2010. I was very grateful to Dr Rhiannon Mason and Dr Areti Galani for inviting me to take part in this stimulating event.

Chapter 4, although subsequently extended, emanated from a seminar organized by the Arts and Humanities Research Council (AHRC) and the Nuffield Council on Bioethics in March 2011. This followed the report on ethics by the Nuffield Council on Bioethics, which features in a number of the chapters of this book. I am grateful to Professor Alistair Burns, who chaired the seminar, and to Hugh Whittall and Katherine Wright from the Nuffield Council who invited me to the seminar and who have continued to encourage me in various ways. Chapter 5 was originally a paper presented at a meeting of the Philosophy Special Interest Group of the Royal College of Psychiatrists, which was held in Aberdeen in October 2011. I am very grateful to Dr John Callender for his tremendous organization of this wonderful event, which was in honour of Professor Eric Matthews. Anyone reading this chapter will recognize my substantial intellectual debt to Professor Matthews, to whom I remain extremely grateful. Chapter 6, which I have again rewritten to a great extent, is based on a talk at another extremely enjoyable and stimulating symposium held at Birmingham University in 2002 organized by Professor Donna Dickenson, whose own work has often inspired me to thoughts that I might not have had otherwise. At the same conference, Professor Christopher Heginbotham was also speaking about capacity. I benefited from his ideas and I am delighted that we have been able to combine our thoughts in a recently published chapter (Hughes and Heginbotham 2013). Chapter 7, with much rewriting, was based on an article that first appeared in *Elderly Client Adviser* (see Acknowledgements). Chapter 8 was originally a paper delivered at the Annual Conference of the Royal College of Psychiatrists in 2004 in Harrogate. I should record here my debt to Charlotte Emmett, from Northumbria University, who was speaking in the same session at that conference and who has over recent years added considerably to my understanding of the notion of decision-making capacity. Chapter 9 is slightly modified from a chapter written for *Les Cahiers de La Fondation Médéric Alzheimer* which appeared in June 2006 (see Acknowledgements). I presented an earlier version of Chapter 10 to the Applied Philosophy Interest Section (APIS) which meets three times a term in Newcastle under the guiding hands of Dr Mary Midgley and Michael Bavidge. My debt to Mary and to Michael will be apparent in these pages, as it is also to Ian Ground and the other members of APIS for their helpful critical comments and intellectual sustenance. My understanding of pain in dementia has been greatly enhanced by the work I did with Doctors Alice Jordan and Claud Regnard and my debt to them is apparent in Chapter 10 too. Chapter 11 is a modified version of a talk I gave in February 2010 on the Advanced European Bioethics course in the Radboud University Nijmegen Medical Centre, where I was afforded a good deal of hospitality, in particular by Dr Wim Dekkers, whose work has also been an inspiration. I was delighted to meet Dr Jenny van der Steen on that occasion. Her work and the work of her colleagues has been and remains seminal in the field of palliative care for people with dementia and I have been delighted to collaborate with Jenny and with Professor Cees Hertogh over the last few years. Chapter 12 derives from a paper presented at the conference entitled 'European Perspectives on End of Life Decision-Making', held at the University of Liverpool in September 2005. I was grateful to Dr Samantha Halliday from the University's Law School for the invitation. In thanking people it is difficult for me not to mention Dr Stephen Louw and Professor Steve Sabat, who have both – throughout the whole of the period covered by this work – been kind friends, supportive of my career and wise intellectual foils.

I am delighted that Ashley McCormick has been willing to join me as a co-author in Chapter 13. We participated together in a Sciart project on 'Memory and Forgetting' back in 2002–2003, which was inspiring for me and enjoyable. The chapter is a reflection on the work that we did together. The original conception for the project came, once again, from Dr Tom Shakespeare, who was at PEALS in Newcastle, but is now at the University of East Anglia. PEALS helped to support the event in conjunction with the Northern Print Studio and the Hatton Gallery at Newcastle University. We owe a great debt of gratitude to the people with dementia and their family or other carers who participated so willingly and generously in their support of the project. The project was funded by the Sciart Consortium and the Arts Council of England. It was a wonderful experience and amongst its many benefits was that it brought me into contact with Tatsumi Orimoto who has generously supported this current work (see Acknowledgements). The penultimate chapter appears as it was originally conceived in 2011 as a short work to celebrate a 'significant' birthday of John Killick, whose work has done so much to encourage the possibility that people might live well with dementia. I was very grateful to Kate Allan, John's collaborator over a good few years, for inviting me to produce the paper for John's birthday. As the Acknowledgements show, I am grateful to John for allowing me to reproduce the paper, which includes some of the poetry that he has composed with people with dementia.

I shall keep my further thanks brief in the hope that those on whom I have relied, or on whom I still rely, know they have my sincere gratitude. I must, however, thank the staff at Jessica Kingsley for their advice and help, in particular my editors Rachel Menzies and Sarah Minty, for their support and patience. Lindsay Turner, my secretary, has provided administrative support, as well as good humour despite hours of typing, for all of which I shall remain extremely grateful. The clinical teams in which I work remain a source of inspiration, not only at Tynemouth Court (our unit for people with severe dementia and behaviours that others find challenging, led by Jill Common), but also our two teams of nurses who work into the nursing and residential care homes in North Tyneside and who also provide a service to those whose behaviour is regarded as challenging. These teams won the *Nursing Times* annual award for community nursing in 2013, deservedly, and I am delighted to work with them: Aileen Beatty, Claire Carss, Susan Gilfoyle, Vikki James, Joan Lowerson, Steven Pearson and Jeanette Shippen.

Throughout, my immediate family has provided the stable base from which I have been able to work; in addition, they have in a variety of ways challenged my thinking and writing, always helpfully. They (Anne, Oliver, Emma and Luke) have my love and affection as ever. So, too, have my parents: both my mother, who somehow manages to combine an active social life and work for the charity *Mind in Croydon* in a manner which would leave many younger people exhausted, and my father, who died in 2011, but who remains a significant influence in our lives. The book is dedicated to his sister, my aunt, who must surely be an example of good ageing in so many ways. One of my enduring memories will always be that of saying goodbye to her at Amsterdam airport, just after she had finished being superior general of her order, as she set off to take up a new post in South Africa, where she was to be supporting and teaching teachers working in many of the poorer parts of the country. The remarkable thing was that she set off to take up this new post in her seventies and did not give it up until her eighties. We all continue to benefit from her sage advice, support and friendship.

Introduction

There are two motivations behind this book. The first is the need to clarify thinking about dementia and about dementia care. These are exciting times for dementia, both in terms of research and in terms of practice. So, for instance, we constantly hear of new scientific advances and, at the same time, there is increasing interest in the many different ways in which the lives of people with dementia can be enhanced by attention to their psychosocial environments. Dementia has even been the topic of conversation, in 2013, at a recent summit of the G8 countries. In the UK, the prime minister, David Cameron, has named dementia the Prime Minister's Challenge. There are more and more examples of ways in which it is possible, as advocated in the report of the Nuffield Council on Bioethics (2009), *Dementia: Ethical Issues*, for people with dementia to live well. Despite the excitement, however, dementia remains a condition which many people fear and the reality for many is that care is sub-optimal. Under these circumstances – of possibility and of concern – it is important that we think clearly about the basics of care. But the basic foundations are philosophical, where clarification of concepts becomes important. The key concepts with which this book is concerned are those of ageing itself, personhood, capacity and best interests, and the nature of care, where this is conceived to be mainly palliative.

The second motivation, which follows from the first, is the wish to make conceptual clarification – the job of philosophy – accessible to those who live with dementia: people who have dementia, their family carers and friends, as well as those who care for them in a variety of professional ways. Philosophical scholarship is daunting to the uninitiated. The aim of this book is to allow people on the front line to engage with the thoughts and arguments that, in any case, underpin their day-to-day experience of dementia. Dementia is associated with ageing: what are the implications of this? People speak of person-centred care in dementia: but what is personhood? Doesn't the person disappear as dementia worsens and, if not, how is personhood maintained? Before almost any decision is now made for a person with dementia there has to be an assessment of the person's capacity or competence. What is this about and how does it link, first, to the underpinning notion of personhood and, second, to broader worries about how the person is cared for as a human being? How should we think of the role of law in relation to the care of older people? And what are our models for understanding care? Is palliative care the best way to think of dementia care and, if so, what are the consequences of this view? In this connection, how are the ethical issues that face us at the end of life, especially in dementia, to be considered? Finally, above all else, given the seriousness of these questions, is there a way to think of dementia that gives us some hope?

To summarize, the book moves from discussion of ageing to consideration of the notion of personhood. I then consider the legal notions of capacity or competence, along with the related themes of best interests, and I touch upon deprivation of liberty. Thoughts about care for the person with dementia lead to reflections on the nature of palliative and supportive care for the person with dementia. I conclude with two essays on art in connection with dementia.

Let me sketch the narrative of the book in more detail to demonstrate the threads that run through the storyline. I start with questions about ageing. These are broad questions about the significance of our lives, especially the significance of our final years. It seems to me that understanding our final years provides some sort of perspective on the whole of our lives. But this does require that we take a broad view. Taking this broad view of ageing suggests that ageing research must also adopt the broad perspective: not only do we wish to add years to life, but (perhaps more importantly) we wish to add life to years. Part of the reason for starting with the notion of ageing is because the context for thinking about dementia has to be thinking about the broader issues. The paradigm of ageing helps to establish the broader view relevant to dementia and research on dementia. In my view, much of this research should be concerned, not only with the psychosocial aspects of care, but also with the philosophical and ethical issues that arise in connection with ageing and dementia. We need, that is, to be thinking about politics and economics as well as sociology when we think about dementia and ageing. But the real political issue concerns how we should be looking after people with dementia *right now*. It often seems that we, as societies, care more about other issues than actually how we might care *for* and care *about* people with dementia, especially in the final stages of dementia. It might be that we would learn something by looking backwards to the ways in which communities cared historically for those in their 'dotage'.

We might be inclined to think that this is all very well, but that dementia is mainly about memory loss and memory loss is mainly a function of the brain. The biomedical approach is certainly helpful in terms of understanding what is happening in the brain during dementia. From a philosophical perspective, however, it is possible to argue that the mind, with which we do our thinking and which we use to remember things, is not just in the head, but extends beyond our brains. So memory loss is not solely a matter of brain dysfunction. Instead, even in thinking about memory, we have to start thinking broadly to the ways in which the mind is external, that is shared between people, which gives us the possibility that others can help to sustain me even if I am entering my 'dotage'. In fact, the theory about the externality of mind helps to set up a broader understanding of what it is to be a person.

Rather than personhood simply depending on something that occurs in the head, it can now be seen as a situated phenomenon. We are situated embodied agents. One consequence of this way of thinking is that our personhood can be held by others. Memory, too, can be held by others as well as by artefacts, by ceremonies, by music and artistically. Once again, it is the broad view of the person which is important and which underpins many of our ethical decisions. The situated embodied agent view of the person, which I shall describe, gives us grounds for arguing that personhood persists even into the terminal stages of dementia. In which case, care at the end of life for people with dementia should be broadly conceived.

What it is for me to be the person that I am is intimately connected to my body. But even this should not be thought of as simply a biomechanical entity occupying physical space. Instead, my body is the way that I interact with the world. It has a certain significance or meaning. It is through the body that we show care; but the body is not just an objective reality, because it is – at the same time – the realization of my subjectivity. Our bodies encapsulate our dreams and aspirations, our hopes and fears, our understanding of the world and our ability to communicate with others. The body is, as it were, more than just the body. It is the means by which my world, including my world of others, exists.

If, therefore, we have a broad view of ageing and dementia, which sits alongside the broad view of personhood or selfhood, it follows that in our dealings with real people we should think broadly. We should not, that is, reduce interactions with other human beings to tick boxes or simple formulae. This is particularly the case when the decisions are of huge importance. Therefore, our judgements about 'mental' decision-making capacity must also be viewed in a broad light. The underlying issue is to do with decision-making and decision-making involves the whole person. There are legal reasons to take a fairly strict view of what it is to have the capacity to make a decision, but we need to think more broadly of competencies in the real world that allow the person to act in and on that world. Judgements about capacity, therefore, must be made from this broad perspective. A narrow legalistic view of capacity may restrict it to a cognitive ability, but the broader view of decision-making brings in values and volitions as we act in and on the world that we inhabit. The implications of making judgements about capacity are very broad, having significant ethical and political ramifications. Although these judgements are usually made one-to-one, they reflect our standing in the larger civic body, where we are required to act under law as civilized individuals, but where we are also affected by social, ethical and political concerns.

In looking after people with dementia, health and social care professionals will inevitably make judgements that can be contested. But the weight of the body politic and the law should not bear down too heavily on people who are, after all, only trying to show solidarity with those who are less fortunate which could be considered a cornerstone of civil society. We are required, after all, to do the best we can for those for whom we should care as fellow citizens. Laws around capacity and incapacity are enacted against a background in which values and moral standards must already be in place. The complexities surrounding incapacity are also demonstrated when this is set alongside notions of mental disorder and mental illness. We can quickly find ourselves trapped in a quagmire of overlapping concepts and blurred boundaries. This should, however, have been predictable because of the complexity of the background that sits behind these apparently simple concepts. Instead, we are always dealing with complexity. Clarity comes from seeing that not only are the facts complicated, but there are also values to be considered at every level. It is because values can be diverse that practice becomes complicated. Recognizing this, however, turns our attention to the importance of communication.

We communicate in many different ways. Communication forms the basis of our relationships and will help to determine whether those relationships are caring or not. As persons we are situated in the worldly context of values, but of course the world contains much more than just facts and values. It also involves our relationships, our emotions and our aesthetic appreciation of life. Again, simply to focus on cognitive mental attributes, which are impaired in dementia, is to lose sight of the broader view of what it is to be a human being engaging in the world. Our human consciousness is much more than self-consciousness. For our consciousness is also consciousness of other people in the world with whom we share our being and with whose minds we interact in public spaces. The models we use to understand people, including people with dementia, therefore, require this breadth of view.

This is seen even when we focus on one particular type of behaviour, such as pain. There is no single sign or symptom that solely depicts pain. Instead, we have to rely on intuition based on our tacit understanding of meaning and significance in the human world. Again, this comes from our shared meanings, from the ways in which our mental lives and subjectivities are not bounded by our skins. Clinical judgements, therefore, must represent a whole way of being and interacting with the world.

We understand significance and we understand the world through the practices that constitute our being-in-the-world. But our patterns of practice can be either virtuous or vicious, so we need to compare them to some sort of horizon which might allow us to deal with the world in a coherent manner on the basis of something, some notion of goodness for instance, which will provide us with surety in our judgements. The underpinning of our patterns of practice provides the basis for our judgements that some actions are right and some are wrong. At the end of life in dementia a variety of moral dilemmas can arise, many of which will be dealt with in a practical manner. But the practices are themselves a reflection of ethical decisions that certain ways of being in the world make sense and allow coherence within our lives. We can, accordingly, agree on the objectives that might characterize good quality care for people with dementia at the ends of their lives. We can talk in terms of models and pathways, which might be helpful, but at root the thing that is at issue is how we meet other people as persons situated in our complex world of facts and values.

It is partly our situated nature that means we cannot be regarded as independent atoms. Rather, we interact so that my being affects your being. And in the final stages of dementia the ability to interact with the person requires that we take the broadest possible view. The broad view of the mind as external entails that judgements about intentions should not solely be based on descriptions of what has been going on in the person's head. The intentional nature of an action can be seen in the action itself. So actions which, by their nature, show that the intention has as its aim the ending of a human life must be regarded with concern, given that the prohibition on intentional killing has been regarded as a cornerstone of civil society.

These reflections, in particular the emphasis on the broad perspective, are supported by an aesthetic view of the world. From art we learn the importance of context, we learn about concepts, about meaningful content and about the concern that characterizes our being with others. Art allows us to wonder. It should encourage our enquiry. It allows us to see everyday objects in a more meaningful light. Art, that is, encourages a broader, more humanistic view of how we might engage with people with dementia in the world. Dementia itself is a concept, but one which relies heavily upon the social constructions that surround it. Once again, the importance of values comes into play. But so, too, does the importance of our mutual inter-dependence. The conceptual and emotional difficulty that we can face, and the ethical dilemmas that we come across, mean that the correct human response, when thinking about dementia, is solicitude. For, there are uncertainties about the world which we must negotiate, including the uncertainties about how we shall die. These cannot be settled merely by appeal to facts. Instead there must be an emotional and sensual or aesthetic human response to our predicament as human beings-in-the-world. Our interconnectedness and solicitude, which can be shown through joy and love and the delight of shared engagement, should underpin the care given to people with dementia. This needs to be achieved at a societal level, where we all have the potential to demonstrate solidarity manifest both by what we say and what we do. In summary, this is the story of what follows.

PART I

Ageing

CHAPTER 1

Our Changing Expectations of Life

What Do We Really Want?

Almost one hundred years ago, in 1922, the play *The Makropulos Affair*, written by a leading Czech writer of the time, Karel Čapek (1890–1938), was first performed in Prague. Almost immediately it was picked up by the composer Leoš Janáček (1854–1928), who turned it into a three-act opera of the same name (*Věc Makropulos*). The opera was first performed in 1926. Unlike Janáček's other operas, such as *The Cunning Little Vixen* or *Katya Kabanova*, *The Makropulos Affair* is not often performed.

The story of *The Makropulos Affair* is, in brief, that 300 years ago the Emperor Rudolf II asked his alchemist, Hieronymus Makropulos, to come up with a potion to extend his life. The potion was tested on Makropulos's daughter, Elina, who fell into a coma, but recovered and ran off with the formula for the potion. She became a famous singer and then spent the next 300 years being the same age, singing, but constantly having to change her name and character so that no one caught on to what was happening. In the opera, Elina, who is now called Emilia Marty (in fact she is always called by names with the letters EM), gets caught up in a law case in which *she* knows all the answers because *she* was involved in what had happened about 100 years before. So, she eventually has to reveal all, but she decides that being perpetually young is boring and distressing, hence she determines to allow death to come naturally and rapidly becomes over 300 years old –

which may be why the opera is not often performed! She dies and the secret Makropulos formula is destroyed.[1]

The Makropulos Affair raises a question about longevity, namely: do we really want it? I suppose the question is, more precisely, for most of us (apart from those who wish to be frozen so they can live for ever), how *much* longevity do we want? Most of us want to live a good long life, but not *too* long. Hence, given that our expectations of life have and are changing, what do we really want?

In this chapter I shall consider the *significance* of the final years. And my argument will be as follows:

- Something has a significance because of its context, or surround.

- The final years are surrounded by the rest of life and by death.

- This implies two things: first, that the final years have to be seen, not in isolation, but in the context of the earlier years and, second, that the inevitability of death also provides the significance of the final years.

- But this means that our understanding of the final years gives us our perspective on life as a whole, including our perspective on death.

- So it does seem important to see the final years in the correct light.

It would be good, if obnoxious, if I thought I could present the correct light in which we should see the final years. It may be helpful to understand why this would be obnoxious. A corollary of my argument would be that presenting you with the correct light in which to see the final years would be to present you with a perspective on life as a whole: I would be telling you how to

---

1   In relating the tale of *The Makropulos Affair*, it is almost impossible not to record the tragically ironic story of poor Richard Versalle, the famous tenor who was singing in the opera in early 1996. On the opening night at the Metropolitan Opera in New York, only a few minutes into Act 1 he had to climb a 20-foot ladder. Having sung the line: 'Too bad you can only live so long' he suffered a heart attack, fell off the ladder and died on stage.

live your lives. That is something we normally leave to people such as our religious leaders or to people of patent goodness and wisdom. Our conversations about ageing are not solely about old age, they are about living the whole of our lives – about living our human lives in the world. This reflects, of course, the prosaic, but nonetheless fascinating, point that we are ageing from soon after conception. In which case, if ageing is really about the whole of life, about living generally, and if – as the philosopher Ludwig Wittgenstein (1889–1951) once noted – in life we are surrounded by death,[2] then (paradoxically) our *lives* are really about dying, at least in terms of significance.

I shall start with the idea that something has a significance because of its context, or surround. The word 'significance' suggests meaning. Indeed, one theory of meaning, of the way in which words stand for objects, is in terms of their signification. We could say that words are signs for objects. Such a theory, however, is generally regarded now as being too simplistic. Instead, philosophers, following Wittgenstein amongst others, would tend to understand meaning in terms of use, or better still in terms of practice. According to this line of thought, to grasp a meaning is to grasp or to have a pattern of practice (a notion to which I shall return in Chapter 11). A meaningful statement can be squared with, it is part of, a practice that in itself makes some sense. The practice is *the given*, within which our utterances have a place. So, significance is to do with meaning and meaning is to do with being situated in a practice – what Wittgenstein also called a 'form of life'.[3] And a form of life is not something on its own: it has many parts, so that other parts surround each component part. A form of life is a whole context of significance.

To return to ageing, the significance of the final years must be judged by the context or surround. Harry Lesser (2006) talked about the 'boundedness' of life. Our final years are bounded too,

---

2   'If in life we are surrounded by death, so too in the health of our intellect we are surrounded by madness' (Wittgenstein 1980, p.44).

3   'the *speaking* of language is part of an activity, or of a form of life' (Wittgenstein 1968, §23); later he goes further and says, 'What has to be accepted, the given, is – so one could say – *forms of life*' (Wittgenstein 1968, p.226)

by the past as by the future. He pointed to two consequences of boundedness being an essential feature of our identity as persons. First, it means that it is part of our identity that we probably decline and certainly die. This is not to deny, on his view, that this is a misfortune and distressing, but, he says, 'decline is part of being a person, not ceasing to be one' (Lesser 2006, p.59). Second, he highlights the relationship to the future, as to the past, and the way in which this relationship is changing with time, because change is an inevitable concomitant of our boundedness. Time, indeed, as some philosophers have said, is a measure of change. It is the notion of the inevitability of change in our lives that *The Makropulos Affair* tempts us to deny.

To summarize:

- something has a significance because of its context, or surround

- the final years are surrounded by the rest of life and by death.

Well, but might we wish to argue that this is simply an empirical, contingent matter, that death is not inevitable? I can think of two immediate responses. First, that an unbounded life, a life like this one but forever, is not something of which we have any real current conception. Many of our day-to-day concepts would have to change in order to understand such an eternal being. How would we, for instance, expect them to behave morally? If you knew you were going to live forever, what would be your attitude towards relationships? What would be your interest in intellectual activity? In other words, the conception of our lives – but our lives lived forever – is not a conception of *our* lives; it is a conception of lives, which are not ours, that we do not understand.

Second, a related response is the one given by the philosopher Bernard Williams (1929–2003) in his essay entitled 'The Makropulos case: Reflections on the tedium of immortality' (Williams 1973). He says that the supposed contingencies – he means things such as decline and death – are not really contingencies at all. He argues,

that an endless life would be a meaningless one; and that we could have no reason for living eternally a human life. There is no desirable or significant property which life would have more of, or have more unqualifiedly, if we lasted forever. In some part, we can apply to life Aristotle's marvellous remark about Plato's Form of the Good: 'nor will it be any more good for being eternal: that which lasts long is no whiter than that which perishes in a day'. (Williams 1973, p.89)

There is nothing about life in itself, in terms of the quantity of life, that adds to the quality of life. The significance of our final years – if meaning comes from quality – may be contained in just *one* aspect of our lives as they are then lived (from our love of music, say, or from a particular relationship).

Williams goes on to say (where EM stands for the various names of Elina Macropulos over the centuries):

The more one reflects to any realistic degree on the conditions of EM's unending life, the less it seems a mere contingency that it froze up as it did. That it is not a contingency, is suggested also by the fact that the reflections can sustain themselves independently of any question of the character that EM had; it is enough, almost, that she has a human character at all. (pp.90–91)

What we sense in the life of Elina Makropulos, or Emilia Marty, is a life of futility and boredom, which are not mere contingent features of her particular character and life, because *any way* we can think to eliminate such features entails eliminating her life qua human life. It would then be a form of life of which we have little comprehension (even if we have some). And the reason for the tedium is precisely that her life is not bounded. The significance of the final years, then, is partly because these are the years during which our boundedness becomes more manifest. Karl Jaspers (1883–1969), the German psychiatrist and philosopher, referred to death as a 'limit situation'. Of course, we come face to face with the limit situation at many points in our lives (every death, every sadness even), but during the final years it is – whether we like it or not, face it or not – a pervasive feature. The inevitability of death provides the significance of the final years.

I have not made so much of the other side of our boundedness, which is that the final years also connect to our earlier lives. Part of the significance or meaning of the final years comes from the narrative that has gone before. Charles Taylor, the Canadian philosopher, once asserted that a basic condition of making sense of ourselves is, 'that we grasp our lives in a *narrative*' (Taylor 1989, p.47). For Taylor, human persons as selves, '…exist only in a certain space of questions, through certain constitutive concerns… And what is in question is, generally and characteristically, the shape of my life *as a whole*' (Taylor 1989 p.50). The extent to which this is true is the extent to which our understanding of the final years fashions our perspective on life as a whole, which includes the meaning of death in our lives. Just as the meaning of a word cannot be grasped in abstraction without the embedding context of a practice or form of life, so too the meaning or significance of my final years is not just what happens then, for it is situated in the narrative of my whole life, which did or did not have this-or-that direction, was or was not entwined with the lives of a loving family, is or is not underpinned by values that remain of importance to me.

Thus,

- the final years have to be seen, not in isolation, but in the context of the earlier years; and the inevitability of death also provides the significance of the final years

- but this means that our understanding of the final years gives us our perspective on life as a whole, including our perspective on death

- so it does seem important to see the final years in the correct light.

To conclude, I shall sketch some features of the final years that I see as important.

First, we need to remember that the view from old age is just different to that of a younger age. In an editorial in the journal *International Psychogeriatrics*, Dan Blazer pondered on the paradox that the frequency of late life depression in the community is lower relatively when compared to the frequency in the young and middle-aged, despite the fact that we might guess that older people are at greater risk of depression because of a mixture of biological, psychological and social factors, from changes affecting the ageing brain to the accumulation of social losses that comes with age (Blazer 2010). Blazer hypothesizes that there may be three psychosocial protective factors: older people 'de-emphasize future planning and prioritize goals which are emotionally meaningful in the present'; older people acquire wisdom; older people are better able to manage stressful life events, because these are expected in this context, they are the stuff of the surroundings of the final years.

These reflections are important, I think, partly because they remind us not to stigmatize older people on the basis of our own perspectives, which simply do not have the benefit of age. The Newcastle philosopher, Michael Bavidge, has made a similar point in cautioning against the possibility of pathologizing old age:

> The thought that human consciousness emerges, develops, and ages should remind us not to pathologize old age…there are mixed costs and benefits attending all stages of life. It is only when these become dysfunctional that we should start treating them as pathological symptoms. We should think of old age as offering alternative rather than impaired ways of experiencing life. (Bavidge 2006, p.49)

Second, there is the importance of our inter-dependence, which becomes more obvious in the final years, but is nonetheless present in all of our lives. Thus, the importance of family, friends, community, social support and so on.

Third, there emerge new ways of *being* in the final years. I have in mind two aspects: there is the aspect of *moment to moment being* and, therefore, the importance of what I am doing right now, of how I am interacting or not, and there is the aspect of *care*, which is required in the final years, which is bodily care, but is also psychological, emotional and spiritual care. Of course, the reality of care as part of the human condition springs from our inter-dependence. But it has deep roots. The philosopher Martin Heidegger (1889–1976), for instance, used the notion of solicitude to describe the way in which we inter-relate as beings of this kind, who have a particular sort of significance for each other (Heidegger 1962, p.158). The significance of *your* final years is – or should be – of significance to *me* because of our mutual standing as human beings, as beings in the world of this type. This aspect of our being underpins the human reaction of care or solicitude: this is why we wash you in this way, why we still talk of your dignity, why we still speak to you and hold your hand.

Fourth, there are the persisting signs of our humanity. Barbara Pointon has written of her husband's life with dementia and of his death. These were her reflections even in the midst of Malcolm's final years:

> Malcolm is surrounded by love. We reach out to communicate with him at a profound level – often through eye contact and gentle whispering and touch – and from him there flows a deep childlike trust, luminosity and reciprocating love – as though it were his very self, the self he was born with, that we are privileged to glimpse... Does it matter what we call it – spirit, soul, inner self, essence, identity – so long as we have experienced it? (Pointon 2007, p.119)

In Barbara's view:

> To stand stripped of everything the world values and to see each other as we really are is a very precious and humbling experience, and one I would never have encountered were it not for the ravages of dementia. (p.119)

It would seem, then, that even in the midst of extreme frailty, there is still the possibility of significance or meaning. In my work with people in the last stages of severe dementia, this has often been my experience, confirmed by the attitudes and accounts of those, like Barbara, who are closest to the person concerned. It is possible, however, to insist that we go beyond the point at which there seems to be any human response at all and ask whether, even here, there is still some semblance of significance. Does human life always have meaning? Are not some lives so devastated by a disease such as dementia that they cannot be regarded as meaningful?

That question impels us towards the demand for active voluntary euthanasia or physician-assisted suicide. For now I shall only say that the *significance* of the final years should not be reduced simplistically to a question about the right to die. However, if we acknowledge that the final years can be characterized as a time of suffering and decline, the spirit of the age (the *Zeitgeist*) is to think about the right to choose death. So I shall return to this issue specifically in Chapter 12.

For now, however, I wish to return to the discussion of the significance of the final years. We should consider Heidegger and the importance of Being. Heidegger (1962) was concerned by the idea of Being (or existence) as such, of our Being as human beings and of what this entails. Raising the existential question (about our existence or being itself), which Heidegger's work does, transcends the *causal* account of our lives as they move from conception to death. Instead we are faced by what Charles Taylor was speaking of when he said that our lives exist 'through certain constitutive concerns'. Our lives, including the lives of moribund human beings, raise questions. For even the moribund have histories: narrative lives constituted by meaning and the possibility of meaning, lives of significance. The frail human body that precariously hangs on to life signifies something. And the something is picked up in a reciprocal way by those who care. The significance of the final years is summed up for me in terms of our mutual embeddedness in the human world of meaning – but this is not just the significance of our final years, it is the significance of our lives.

What might we *really* want given our changing expectations of life? I would vote for something that we have *always* wanted, along the lines of Heidegger's notion of solicitude, but perhaps in a more settled manner, without the anxiety that attended Heidegger's concerns about Being: the experience of authentic human love.

CHAPTER 2

Research, Ageing and Dementia

Introduction

In this chapter I wish to suggest that research into ageing is the best paradigm for dementia research. But I shall need to explain what I mean by this and why, indeed, I am saying it. To anticipate, elsewhere in the chapters that follow I shall frequently argue that we need a broad view, in particular a broad view of the person. This will affect our ethical judgements, but also our judgements about models and how to provide care. Similarly, here my argument is that we need a broad view of research and research that allows a broad view (even if it is itself detailed). The imperative of the broad view is, I shall argue, an ethical imperative.

Research into ageing, which I shall now refer to as ageing research (although the research itself is often young!), is as it states. It involves any research into ageing itself: into the mechanisms of ageing at a biological level, into the psychological or physical manifestations of ageing, or into the social aspects of ageing, and so on. It might involve demographic studies, economic analysis, issues to do with housing and transport, understanding of volunteerism, as well as research into genetics and telomere length (telomeres are at the ends of the strands of our chromosomes and longer telomeres have been associated with better ageing), or nutrition, or the mechanisms of cell death and so forth. In order really to understand ageing research, however, it is useful to contrast it with related fields of research.

Cancer researchers, for instance, will often be interested in the same issues as those who work in ageing research, such as genetics, nutrition and cell death. But the cancer researcher is asking how the changes observed relate to cancer. The researcher into ageing, meanwhile, may be interested in the fact that a particular change leads to cancer, but will also be interested in the possibility that the selfsame change or observation, of telomere length for instance, might be relevant to dementia or to frailty in general and so on. Another researcher may be looking at stem cells in the gut to say something about bowel cancer, whereas ageing research is interested in stem cells because of what they might tell us about ageing in general, which will involve a variety of age-related diseases, from bowel cancer to Parkinson's disease to osteoarthritis. This is not the place to give further insights into the nature of ageing research, even if I were able to do so, but I shall briefly discuss possible aims of ageing research.

The aims of ageing research

Well, one aim might be longevity. Indeed, ageing research is certainly interested in longevity because, by studying species or individuals within species that live long lives it is possible to hypothesize about the biological mechanisms of ageing. Indeed, research specifically looking at longevity has produced a wealth of findings generating numerous theories and deeper understanding of the processes involved (Gray, Proctor and Kirkwood 2013).

But most people would accept, including most researchers into ageing, that quantity of life without quality of life does not seem to be a helpful outcome. More than that, it is the outcome that many people dread and it can be regarded as a downside of modern medicine if people are kept alive to suffer longer. Of course, there is a big jump to be made from biological research into ageing to clinical practice. I shall come to this shortly. But if the biological research were only fuelling the tendency to keep people alive (as many older people say, 'beyond my sell-by date') then its usefulness would be highly questionable.

The relationship, however, between quantity and quality is complex. It might be, for instance, that as we understand more about how and why people live longer we might learn more about how to improve the quality of life. The earlier discussion about the difference between those researching into ageing and those researching into cancer and other age-related diseases is part of the issue. It might be that too narrow a focus on specific diseases will miss the important underlying point, which is that many of these diseases are fundamentally related to ageing and that ageing itself must be understood. Of course, in fact, many researchers looking at specific conditions are aware of this and they will, accordingly, think quite broadly about the aspects of the biology they are otherwise focusing on. This does not detract from the point, however, that there may be more fundamental issues to do with ageing which, if we understood them properly, would help us to combat different aspects of age-related diseases (Kirkwood 2008).

The exciting idea is that we could see the 'rectangularization', or squaring off, of the morbidity curve, as depicted in Figure 2.1.

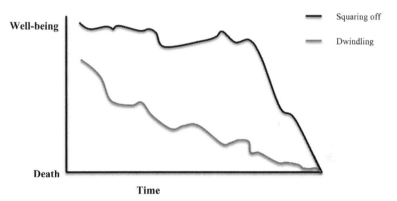

Figure 2.1 Squaring off the morbidity curve

Figure 2.1 shows, in the bottom line, the sort of trajectory that many people fear, namely the slow but steady loss of functions and capabilities over a long period of time, which has been called 'dwindling'. What most of us would prefer, as shown in the top line of Figure 2.1, is that we should live a full and contented life for as long as possible and then die really quite quickly over a matter of days rather than weeks and months. The hope is that, as we understand more about ageing, we shall be better placed to cope with age-related diseases so that our lives can be fuller even into the extremes of old age.

This aspiration, it turns out, is not a castle in the sky. There is evidence that dying occurs more quickly than it once did, in the sense that people are able to function and enjoy life for longer and closer to the point of death. Again, however, there is some complexity here. A series of important papers have emerged from the Newcastle 85+ Study, which looked at 1042 people born in 1921 and living in Newcastle upon Tyne and North Tyneside. One very interesting finding has been that, although on average the people over 85 had 4.5 diseases each, they still rated their overall health as good, very good or excellent compared to others of the same age (Collerton *et al.* 2009). Hence, although age-related diseases are common in the older population, they are being lived with in a way that allows many older people still to feel fulfilled and to be content and optimistic. Research into social aspects of ageing (as pursued by social gerontologists for instance) helps us to understand the ways in which, and how, well-being and quality of life are maintained into old age. In other words, it is possible to study quality of life itself, as well as the length of life, but the two things interact.

If quantity and quality are two aims of ageing research, a third might simply be enquiry. After all, we should not undervalue the importance of a basic thirst for knowledge, which is itself a manifestation of human well-being and flourishing. A perfectly reasonable and rational aim of ageing research, that is, might simply be to understand what is going on, whether at the biological level, or in terms of psychology or sociology. One hope is that such basic research, by serendipity, might lead to a major advance or shift in terms of the paradigms that drive and lead research. But even if there is no such breakthrough, painstaking enquiry can still lead, step by step, to greater understanding which can itself be regarded as a good, even if no obvious practical consequences ensue. This thought is counter-cultural, but I would suggest that if we lose the desire for knowledge and understanding *as such*, we lose something in just the same way that human life would be worse off without aesthetic experiences, irrespective of whether those experiences have any tangible benefits beyond the experiences themselves.

Dementia and ageing

There are very good reasons to argue that dementia is not a part of normal ageing. One obvious reason is that most older people do not have dementia. For instance, only 6 per cent of people between the ages of 75 and 79 have dementia; over the age of 95 years 45 per cent have dementia, which means that most people of that age *do not* (Fratiglioni and Qiu 2013). There are also important practical reasons to emphasize that dementia is not part of normal ageing. Many people with dementia and their carers have the experience of seeing their doctors and being told that their worries about memory (or indeed other physical disorders) are unfounded because: 'It's just your age.' This attitude can reasonably be called ageist inasmuch as it denies help to people simply on the basis of their age where they would receive help if they were younger. It may also reflect therapeutic nihilism, that is, the belief that nothing can be done and therefore nothing should be attempted and the person should be encouraged just to accept the facts of life, which in this case are the facts of ageing: as the saying goes, 'Age breeds aches.' So, we wish to make the point quite firmly that dementia is not a matter of normal ageing.

The key word here is 'normal'. It clinches the deal. It seems to establish, beyond argument, that dementia is abnormal. It does this for very good reasons, in that we wish people with dementia to be helped and treated if at all possible. If, however, we remove the word 'normal', the statement that dementia is not a matter of ageing is false. For, as the numbers above demonstrate, dementia is a matter of ageing in that it becomes more prevalent as age increases. There is something about ageing that causes dementia. Not only is this true at the level of epidemiology, where diseases are studied in populations, but it is also true at the biological level. If, for instance, we think of the amyloid plaques and the neurofibrillary tangles that are the most obvious hallmarks of Alzheimer's disease when brains are examined under the microscope, it is again true that these changes in the brain become more prevalent as we age. You would not find many plaques and tangles in the brains of 30 or 40-year-olds.

Now, however, things start to become more confusing, because, in fact, plaques and tangles can be found in younger people and they can be found, sometimes quite obviously, in older people who do not have dementia. In other words, they do not present with the clinical features of dementia, such as memory loss, disorientation, language problems and problems with activities of daily living. The bugbear, therefore, is the word 'normal' when attached to the notion of ageing. For the question that has to be asked is how can the line be drawn between what is and what is not normal ageing?

I do not wish to pursue this point more fully, but it is a topic I have discussed at more length in *Thinking Through Dementia* (Hughes 2011a, pp.19–27). Pursuing this theme elsewhere, I have suggested the slogan 'Dementia is dead, Long live ageing' (Hughes 2013a). In part, this draws on the work of Peter Whitehouse who has argued that, instead of thinking of dementia, we should think in terms of the ageing brain (Whitehouse and George 2008). But, whilst I do not wish to pursue these issues in detail, I shall just make one point, which is that the notion of 'normal' has to be seen as evaluative. In other words, our judgements about what is normal and what is not are value judgements. Surely, it might be said, the pathology defines what is normal and what is not. It is true that there are criteria that can be drawn upon. A certain number of plaques and tangles down the microscope will be counted as signifying Alzheimer's disease, for instance. But what we know is that there will be people with too few plaques and tangles who will nevertheless present clinically as having dementia and there will be people with too many plaques and tangles who, nonetheless, do not appear clinically to have dementia (Snowdon 2003). The truth is that the numbers reflect judgements of value about statistical norms. Thus, most people with this number of plaques and tangles display such and such symptoms and signs and it is judged that this is abnormal. In making that judgement we are saying that the behaviour is not, in some sense, conducive to health or well-being, where those concepts themselves are predicated on evaluative judgements. The importance of values, from diagnosis to treatment, has been established in the seminal work of Bill Fulford (1989).

Nevertheless, to return to the issue of normal ageing, once we grasp that in terms of biology and behaviour there is a continuum, which means that evaluative judgements must be made to determine where normality begins and ends, then the statement that dementia is not part of normal ageing starts to seem conceptually more complex. It is complex because, at the margins, what will and will not count as dementia, and what will and will not count as normal ageing, is not completely certain. At the margins, therefore, it may seem more reasonable to send away an older person with worries about his or her memory with some simple reassurance.

Immediately, there are a number of important caveats that would have to be attached to this statement. First, doctors often think that they are being reassuring – and will sometimes write in the notes 'patient reassured' – when in fact the patient is still extremely worried. So sending someone away with reassurance should not be undertaken lightly and should be accompanied by practical reassurance in the form of actual follow-up or very clear invitations to seek further help if the problems persist or worsen. Second, just because at the margins there may be 'normal' people who could wrongly be described as 'abnormal', this should not be used as an excuse to avoid helping someone who might be helped, if not by treatment, perhaps by advice and psychological or social support. To fail to provide such basic help would be a dereliction of duty on the part of any health or social care professional.

What I hope to have established, despite these caveats, is that dementia and ageing are inextricably linked. I now wish to go further and argue that dementia research must, at its best, take as its paradigm ageing research. In saying this, I am making a supposition about ageing research, which is more or less true, namely that it will tend to take the broad view. Of course, some people like to take a very limited view of what constitutes ageing research, but my point is that, *at a conceptual level*, what we mean by 'ageing' cannot be confined too tightly. Rather, the concept of ageing points outwards towards profound human concerns.

The paradigm of ageing

My suggestion that ageing research is the best paradigm for dementia research is, at one level, easily granted and may, in fact, already be the case. Inasmuch as dementia research is already broad, involving biological, psychological and social models, it is as ageing research should be. Indeed, it may be that dementia research is broader in some respects – it would be difficult and somewhat pointless to try to ascertain whether or not this was so. My intention, however, is to dig to a deeper point and argue that ageing is the better paradigm precisely because, conceptually, its breadth encourages a better perspective on the relevant and important issues. In line with my slogan 'Dementia is dead, Long live ageing', the project I am encouraging entails that we see the term 'dementia' to be otiose, because we do not really know what it points to. Strictly speaking, it points only to a clinical syndrome, to a collection of symptoms and signs. Of course, it points to more than this: to human stories, to battles over nomenclature, to neurophysiology and to increasing frailty, but it is essentially just a syndrome. Moreover, its actual meaning, 'loss of mind', is stigmatizing and removed from the realities of the clinical syndrome. Better, therefore, to regard dementia as part and parcel of ageing (without the contentious use of 'normal') and to think, accordingly, of dementia research as research on ageing. This has the added advantage of compelling ageing to be viewed from the broad perspective, which the reality of (what is referred to as) 'dementia' demands. Not only, therefore, must ageing be considered from biological, psychological, social and even spiritual viewpoints, we must also – in thinking about ageing – consider its ethical and political ramifications, its relevance to technological advances, its demographic and economic implications, as well as the need to consider infrastructure, design and planning with reference to ageing. (The need to think broadly in this way is a theme that recurs, in particular in Chapter 11 when I talk about models and care pathways.) Dementia, too, is a whole community concern, and hence the recent turn in the UK towards the idea of dementia-friendly communities seems utterly appropriate.[4]

There are three types of research: basic, applied and translational. Basic research is concerned with fundamentals. Basic biological research seeks to understand biological processes, for instance, without attempting to put this understanding to any immediate practical use. Biological understanding, for instance, that the levels of the neurotransmitter acetylcholine are lower in the brains of people with Alzheimer's disease, might lead to practical outcomes, such as the development of drugs to decrease the breakdown of acetylcholine in the brain, which have clinical benefits: a modest improvement in cognitive function.[5] Basic biology, by serendipity, might shift the scientific paradigm. But even though this is unlikely to occur (paradigm shifts are not common!), basic research must continue for the reasons expressed previously: the desire to enquire and understand is constitutive for human flourishing.

Applied research, as opposed to basic or 'pure' research, usually aims to use scientific knowledge or theories in order to solve a practical problem of some sort or other. If, for instance, we have a theory of how we might change doctors' decision-making, say about whether or not patients have the capacity to consent or about their best interests, we might devise an intervention (a pro-forma or a care pathway), which we can then put into effect to test its effectiveness. Applied research does not tend to shift the paradigm, because it tends to reflect the current paradigmatic thought. Change follows applied research step by step. But, again, this type of research is very important in that it will (step by step) alter practice and, one would hope, improve it in line with current thinking.

My reason for sketching these types of research is to arrive at the third type, which is very much in vogue, namely translational

---

4   See Department of Health n.d.
5   For more details on the biology and other facts relevant to dementia, please see Hughes 2011b.

research. Indeed, translational research is so much in vogue that it is wise, in seeking funding for research, to 'badge' any research that you do as translational! The idea is that the outcome of research should be swiftly translated from the laboratory to the bedside. The complaint is that, without the translational impetus, basic research simply stays in the laboratory, or at least it remains purely theoretical and it has little impact on the world. The effects of research need to be translated from theory to practice. Translational research aims to get something done more quickly, which seems perfectly sensible.

It also has built into it the possibility of a feedback loop, that once results have been put into effect this should help to generate new problems, which can be tackled theoretically and then practically once again. Participatory action research has this feel, because it seeks real effective change quickly as a result of the participation of people who are actually affected by the condition, in this case dementia.

My interest in this is just to highlight one point. Participatory action research, in my opinion, has things the right way around because it starts with the experience of real people *now* and the real problems they face. It starts with the world. Research that starts in the laboratory, or at least in a purely theoretical manner, is simply unlikely to 'translate' into something that is practical and useful in the world, except by serendipity. My objection is admittedly semantic. I think all we really have here is basic 'pure' research and applied research, and one form of applied research is participatory action research, where real problems drive the experiments, whether they be in the laboratory or in the community, and the experiments lead to action. The translation is unlikely to occur unless the laboratory (whether this be a genetics laboratory or a brain scanner) is already cognizant of the outcomes that are required. In other words, the move is not from the laboratory to the bedside, but from the bedside to the laboratory and back to the bedside. This seems right, and it still allows that basic research should continue because it might be possible that it should interact with applied paradigms and, in addition, there is always the unlikely possibility of a serendipitous breakthrough.

But if all this is accepted, if useful research is likely to start in the world and is to be broadly conceived, because ageing must be broadly conceived, then it follows that our areas of interest should also be broad. To make progress in the field of ageing will often require action, not only in terms of biology or pharmacology, but also in areas that involve public policy, economics, ethics, law and so on. The pull to think broadly, which is a constitutive feature associated with ageing, places dementia research, as a part of the broader paradigm of ageing, in a social and political context of great consequence.

Let me make this more concrete. Dementia is a part of ageing. Ageing raises a host of worldly concerns. We are pulled in the direction of the world and, therefore, towards the concerns of real people in the world. The question for research is: what will help now? Take, therefore, the problem that many people with dementia find it difficult at some point to stay in their own homes, with or without a spouse to care for them, with or without family to support them. What would help now? The answer will often be that 24-hour help at home would go some way towards stabilizing the crises that arise. The reality, of course, is that such 24-hour help, at least in the UK, is usually impossible because it is unaffordable. So how would this be achieved? By economic, technological advances supported by public policy and willpower. Enabling people to stay at home, if that is our aim, will require a broad range of inputs (Treloar and Crugel 2010). But all of this is a long way from the sort of research that often attracts funding. Ageing changes the subject, because it directs our attention elsewhere, away from the laboratory bench to the lived experience of ordinary people. But this ageing paradigm – the broad conceptualization of ageing, which includes dementia – is not the paradigm that governs the perspective of many researchers at present. And this is because the real problems of people *now* are too broadly based to be tackled, unless it be at a political or societal level. The hope, rather, is that lives will be improved by the magic bullet of a drug, or a care pathway, or by an investigation or diagnosis, or by advance care planning. But even if these things will help, the real issue is that of ageing. The real issue is *how we live our lives into old age*. In which case, some of our research should be political, ethical and philosophical as well as biological, psychological and social.

The imperative of ethics

My argument is that, conceptually, understanding ageing is a broad endeavour, but it is the right one. Research into ageing becomes an ethical imperative because how we, individually and as societies, live our lives is of crucial moral concern. I take it that morality is concerned with how we lead good lives, how we live in the right way. To age is to live, and the imperative is that we should do this well, that is in a good or right way, not badly or in the wrong way, for living well is to flourish as a human being, which is surely what we should all wish and aim to do. An immediate link can be made with the requirements of health and social care. The ethical imperative for ageing research partly involves the imperative for good quality health and social care. My suggestion in the previous section is that we need to look at how things are *now* for people with dementia, which will help to determine the direction of research, or the direction of the ethical imperative.

Reflecting, inevitably, my own interests, I shall briefly consider the issue of early diagnosis of dementia and make some comparisons with palliative care. The issue of early diagnosis of dementia has recently become controversial. It used to be said, without controversy, that an early diagnosis was good. More recently people have questioned this. They have asked what the real benefits of an early diagnosis might be given that pharmacological treatments are acknowledged only to be modestly effective and given that the diagnosis is likely to cause worry and anxiety. I shall not try to present all of the arguments on both sides of this debate.

But one argument in favour of early diagnosis, which is sometimes given, is that it allows planning for the future. Even this, however, can be disputed on the grounds that some advance care planning is not particularly realistic in dementia. For instance, statements about where you wish to live when you have severe dementia may simply not be honoured because of practical problems. At an early stage, stipulating in great detail how you wish to be treated medically may also turn out to be irrelevant to the circumstances that arise in actual fact later in your particular case. In other words, your advance refusal of treatment might turn out to be inapplicable. Advocates of advance care planning, however, will retort that there are other elements of planning that seem very sensible, for instance, to think about who will make decisions for you should you become unable to make decisions for yourself, which in England and Wales would be covered by Lasting Powers of Attorney (LPAs), which are a form of proxy decision-making. This seems sensible, but those who are against early diagnosis can respond that this sort of planning should be occurring in any case, whether or not we have dementia. As I write this, for instance, I know that, should I develop dementia, power of attorney for financial matters has already been arranged in favour of my wife and children. So the need for an early diagnosis seems irrelevant.

The arguments about early diagnosis continue on both sides. Of course, a very important argument should be the one which reflects the views of people with dementia themselves and of their carers. When the Nuffield Council on Bioethics consulted over its report, *Dementia: Ethical Issues*, it found that most people wished to know the diagnosis as soon as possible, although some people did not (Nuffield Council on Bioethics 2009, pp.42–5).

So maybe the answer is that whether or not a person is told the diagnosis early should rightly depend on his or her particular views and, therefore, the imperative is that the clinician should use good communication skills in order to elicit the person's real wishes in this regard. Often people wish to know the diagnosis because giving a name to what is happening to them (or to their loved ones) is itself helpful. It immediately provides a framework for understanding. This seems very reasonable. It would be less reasonable if someone wished to have an early diagnosis in the hope that this would lead to very positive advantages of the sort that are contested, because the benefits might not be forthcoming.

The Nuffield Council's Working Party picked up from the Alzheimer's Society the notion of a 'timely diagnosis'. A timely diagnosis reflects the wishes of the person with dementia and his or her carers. The Nuffield Council's report stated:

> Even where there is little doubt about the accuracy of the diagnosis, it cannot be assumed that *every* person with dementia will find that the advantages of early diagnosis and disclosure outweigh the disadvantages. A distinction between 'early' and 'timely' diagnosis is helpful in this respect. As the Alzheimer's Society noted in its response to our consultation: 'for conveying a diagnosis to be helpful and appropriate, it must be timely, with benefits balanced against risks. Where a person stands to be distressed to the point where no benefit can be derived, then even an early diagnosis is perhaps not a timely one'. This approach is in line with our own emphasis on considering both the well-being and the autonomy of the person with dementia: where the person is not seeking a diagnosis, and where their well-being is unlikely to be enhanced by the diagnosis, then it is inappropriate to force that diagnosis upon them. (Nuffield Council on Bioethics 2009, paragraph 3.16)

Now, of course, good clinical judgement will be required to decide when the time is right to give the timely diagnosis. But my feeling is that it is correct to say that the timing will be idiosyncratic. It cannot be dictated ahead of time and must depend on the individual circumstances of those involved.

There is, however, another concern. The original impetus behind the demand for early diagnosis was, and is, the knowledge that many people are not being given the diagnosis when they perhaps should be. There is a great variety of reasons why this happens, from paternalistic attitudes on the part of doctors, to a lack of confidence or knowledge. There does seem to be something wrong with people not being told when they want to be told and should be. So the appeal for early diagnosis seemed quite appropriate. But the deeper concern is that the demand for early diagnosis shifts into a demand for *earlier* diagnosis. That is, the demand starts to be that people should be given the diagnosis as early as possible and even that a 'diagnosis' should be made before 'dementia' has actually started. A rational reason for this can be given, namely that if we can identify the condition before it is manifest, then it might be possible to give treatment before dementia has caused any problems. Hence, we now have the notion of Mild Cognitive Impairment (MCI), which is a pre-dementia state upon which huge amounts of research have been expended. Recently, the notion of MCI has been enshrined in the newest (fifth) edition of the Diagnostic and Statistical Manual (DSM-5) in the guise of Mild Neurocognitive Disorder.[6]

There are, inevitably, worries about MCI, which are recorded in fuller detail elsewhere (Hughes 2006a). One particular worry is that the 'diagnosis' of MCI will itself be stigmatizing and produce anxiety (Bond and Corner 2006).

There is also a larger-scale, more nebulous, but interesting worry that the development of MCI reflects political and economic pressures. So far, there are no treatments for MCI. But if there were to be treatments, even if they were only to produce modest effects, it is highly likely that the drug companies would make massive profits from marketing the products. This, in turn, would be hugely beneficial for the economies of the relevant countries. Meanwhile, researchers in universities who are seeking funding can, therefore, find ready sources of financial support from the pharmaceutical industry. Furthermore, in the UK it is now overtly acknowledged that the government wishes to encourage researchers to participate in industry-led research because this helps to keep those industries in the UK rather than allowing them to go abroad where they can perhaps pursue research in an environment that is more lenient in terms of bureaucracy.

Such comments are often greeted with a degree of derision and can be characterized as paranoid, as showing a naïve belief in conspiracy theory. Nevertheless, research into MCI has shown that its drivers are sociologically complex (Moreira *et al.* 2008). These suggestions would be naïve and paranoid if they were based on the supposition that individuals were meeting and plotting in

6   See American Psychiatric Association 2013.

a cabal-like manner perhaps in dimly lit and smoke-filled rooms! But the suggestion does not have to be of this sort. It is simply the suggestion that there are powerful social, political and economic forces at play, which tend to move our societies in particular directions unthinkingly. These forces may operate below the level of planning. Once certain building blocks are in place, such as the knowledge that many people are not given the diagnosis soon enough, the hope that earlier diagnosis will lead to cure, the concern that there will be unemployment if the pharmacology industry decamps to Poland, an edifice starts to be built in which people must be diagnosed as soon as possible, before the condition even emerges, so that they can be treated and live without dementia.

Moreover, we hear it said in some quarters that there is also an ethical imperative that people should participate in research. Initially it is said that people have a *right* to participate in research, but ethicists emerge suggesting that there is a *duty* to participate in research because we all potentially benefit from the results of research (Harris 2005). So there is an ethical imperative, apparently, that we should all participate in the endeavour that will lead to the absence of dementia.

Now, I would not wish to suggest that all of this is nonsense. But I would wish to suggest that it shows a lack of perspective. It starts to seem as if our lives are to be driven totally by the concerns of biomedicine and industry, for instance. But this is foolishness. The driver behind the construction of the edifice I have described is the view that we can cure dementia and get rid of it from our lives. There are a number of problems with this. For instance, it must quickly be said that dementia is not one single thing. It can even be questioned to what extent Alzheimer's disease is one single thing (Richards and Brayne 2010). My point, however, is that if dementia is part of ageing, albeit not part of normal ageing, then it is likely to remain a feature of our lives unless we can rid our lives of ageing itself. But to age is to live, and to live is to do all sorts of things beyond the realms of biomedicine, which also do not always feed into the economic imperative to preserve or increase the Gross Domestic Product (GDP). We need a broader view.

Well, one thing that the broader view might give us is a view of people who are already suffering from dementia and a view of the sort of help and support that they require *right now*. Much of this, I contend, will be palliative. I shall, later in this book, discuss models of care, including the palliative care model and what I consider to be a broader model, that of supportive care. (In the end, I shall wonder whether we need models at all!)

With this broader perspective in mind, it is interesting to reflect that when the National Dementia Strategy for England was produced in draft form for consultation, although the need for early diagnosis was emphasized and with it the concomitant requirement for memory clinics to be established, there was no reference to the palliative care needs of people with dementia. There was a predictable response to this and the dementia strategy in its final form acknowledges the importance of palliative care. Nevertheless, it is not the palliative care needs of people with dementia that are attracting controversy, but the perceived need for early diagnosis. Whilst funding to establish memory clinics is put in place, the funding to provide palliative care for people with dementia until the ends of their lives is not so evident. There is no similar drive to enable people with dementia to live in their own homes until they die through the provision of large-scale health and social care support on a par with the sort of support provided to memory assessment services and memory clinics. Many people with dementia live in residential and nursing homes and, again, we do not see state funding (which, in any case, is delegated to local authorities) for this sector of the population. Most of the care for people in care homes is provided by too few qualified staff or by underpaid care assistants who are unqualified in a professional sense. Efforts are made to improve the quality of care for people in care homes, but the lack of proper funding and a lack of oversight to produce real quality improvements is noticeable. Despite the hard work and commitment of many who work in this sector, society (often through the media) is quick to point towards and emphasize scandals in terms of care, but not quick to demand that funding be supplied to improve the quality of care beyond the minimal standards that so often obtain.

The ethical imperative, therefore, is that we should have good health and social care right now. Research into ageing, therefore, is an ethical imperative because how we live our lives is of crucial moral concern. Not only should we wish to flourish throughout our lives, including into old age, even if we suffer from illnesses, including dementia, but, in addition, understanding ageing entails understanding the meaning of our lives. Faced by the fact that our lives are bounded, that is that we shall die, questions of meaning become more important perhaps than questions about the causes of disease and the necessity of wealth. This is not to say that seeking causes and the quest for wealth are necessarily bad, but just to highlight that they occur within a context, and the context is one of meaning where the purpose of our lives comes into sharp focus given life's finitude.

The only way around the concerns that I am expressing would be if we could live forever. The problem with that prospect, apart from its unreality, is that it would change things so radically that we would not then know of what we were speaking. It would be hard, that is, to know what might be the meaning of life under such circumstances. Rather than such speculations, however, I would prefer to stick to the life that we know, that is the life in which we age now.

Atavistic tendencies

To complete this chapter, I wish to highlight the benefits of an historical view. My theme has been that we need a broad view of research and research that allows a broad view, as is required by the concept of ageing. Research too finally focused on biomedical causes and driven by the quest for economic success will not provide the correct foundations for research on ageing. Not that causes and wealth-creation are irrelevant or unimportant, but just that they do not provide the full picture. The broader view will, I suggest, take more notice of how things are now, which brings into perspective more clearly the notion of care over against cure.

But this might also make us look back, in an atavistic manner, to the circumstances of our grandparents or great-grandparents. Atavism, looking back to the life of our forebears, might encourage us to think that care in those days was better, in part because people had more of a sense of community. Small communities were prone to look after their older members, even when they were forgetful. Thus, we find in the early-eighteenth century:

> poor relief had served to bind aged dependents to a network of individuals in the community – to poor-law care-givers (be they family or neighbors), individuals who agreed to house them, and, of course, to the members of the vestry whom they saw weekly when they went to collect their pensions or make their new petitions. (Ottaway 2004, p.274)

Susannah Ottaway adds, in her chronicle of old age in England in the 1700s:

> Most of the aged, and even the great majority of the elderly poor remained outside of workhouse walls. The traditional sense that the aged deserved poor relief *within* (not isolated from) their communities remained strong despite the efforts of cynical social critics and overworked local vestries. (p.275)

We see something of this in the poem of 1800 by William Wordsworth (1770–1850), 'The Two Thieves, or The Last Stage of Avarice', in which he describes the little boy and his grandfather (Dan) who go out each day thieving. No one complains, however,

> For grey-headed Dan has a daughter at home,
> Who will gladly repair all the damage that's done;
> And three, were it asked, would be rendered for one.
>
> (Wordsworth 2000, p.217)

In a note written later in his life, Wordsworth said that he observed this pair of thieves when he was a boy at Hawkshead School. 'No book could have so early taught me to think of the changes to which human life is subject…' (Wordsworth 2000, p.699, n. 216).

Old Man! Whom so oft I with pity have eyed,
I love thee, and love the sweet boy at thy side:
Long yet mayst thou live! for a teacher we see
That lifts up the veil of our nature in thee.

(Wordsworth 2000, p.217)

In atavistic mode, then, we might hanker after the good old days! These days, a man in his eighties, seemingly with cognitive impairment ('the lost look of dotage'), who was taking his young grandson out to steal, would certainly be subject to safeguarding proceedings, if not compulsory detention under the Mental Health Act!

Of course, all was not rosy in the old days. Life was harder and shorter for most people. Nevertheless, we might feel that some aspects of life were better, perhaps that the quality of care was better as a consequence of there being closer communities. There may be something in this, although we should not romanticize the past: the picture was variable, as it is today. But this historical perspective at least suggests that we might do better with a perspicuous account. To understand ageing broadly requires all sorts of approaches. Research into ageing requires a broad view, a biopsychosocial view, but also an historical, ethical, spiritual, legal, economic and political perspective. For, to understand ageing, we must understand ourselves and, to understand ourselves fully, we must recognize the extent to which we are persons of significance: persons for whom the world and our lives in it hold meaning. Research on dementia and ageing, therefore, takes place within this broad domain of meaning and significance in which all sorts of things might lift up 'the veil of our nature'.

PART II

Personhood

CHAPTER 3

Memory

Inner or Outer?

Introduction

In this chapter I shall say something about memory loss. I shall say something about clinical aspects of memory loss, but I want to say something about (what could be called) the philosophical underpinnings of memory. These underpinnings inform (or should inform) our clinical encounters with people who have memory difficulties. To anticipate, I want to say that our understanding of memory has a huge amount to do with our understanding of persons. For being a person, including being a person with dementia, is to be a whole lot of things, with a whole lot of ways of engaging with the world and with other people. My argument is that memory is many things and I shall attempt to show some of them. My aim in doing so is to suggest something about our engagement with people with dementia. But, first, we need to think about things that people say about the mind, because our memories are mental: we treasure them (if we do) in our minds.

Causal and constitutive accounts

One of the really crucial things in debates about the mind is to make a distinction between causal and constitutive accounts. For example, there is a lot of effort being put into improving our understanding of consciousness. So, it is quite easy to find papers suggesting that consciousness is this-or-that physical correlate. In other words, researchers get people to think of something – to be conscious of something – and then perform brain scans to show which bits of the brain light up when the person is conscious of whatever it is they have been concentrating on. They conclude that this bit of the brain is where consciousness is: it is the physical bit of the brain that correlates with consciousness. And all of this is undoubtedly true, that consciousness should (in one sense) be physically construed as this-or-that. If this-or-that goes wrong, we shall suffer a loss of consciousness or some sort of disruption to our conscious level.

This sort of research is fine and dandy, but the problem is that such research is typically research concerning the *causal* underpinnings of consciousness. Although the researchers might then argue that consciousness is this-or-that physical thing or event, they have not actually said what consciousness *is*. Instead they have said that when this particular bit of the brain is working the person is conscious of colours, and when that bit is working they are thinking about arithmetic or whatever. This bit causes colour consciousness and that bit causes us to add up correctly. In doing this, they have given a *causal* explanation of consciousness rather than a *constitutive* account, where the constitutive account ought to help us with our deeper understanding of consciousness. The difficulty is that this deeper understanding is likely to be found in the writings of poets, rather than in the writings of neuroscientists. This is problematic, because what we actually need is some sort of understanding that brings together the causal and constitutive accounts and does not leave us with some form of dualism, that is a world in which the two accounts simply cannot meet.

Causal accounts of memory

All of this can then be said of memory too. We need to distinguish between causal and constitutive accounts of memory. Causal accounts will see memory as being closely linked to particular parts of the brain. Thus, for instance, thinking of the very common type of recall memory that is often tested in clinics, whereby you might be given a name and address to remember and then asked the name and address a few minutes later, we know that this sort of recall memory is closely associated with the medial temporal lobe of the brain. In particular, there is a part of the temporal lobe, towards the middle of the brain, called the hippocampus. With modern neuroimaging it is possible to measure the hippocampus quite precisely. It is then possible to show that there is a correlation between loss of recall memory and atrophy or shrinkage of the medial temporal lobe and in particular of the hippocampus. In a condition such as Alzheimer's disease, where this is the obvious sort of memory that is slowly disappearing, it is possible to watch the hippocampus also slowly disappearing.[7] So we can say that the pathology which affects the hippocampus causes memory loss and, by implication, this sort of memory must be located (in some sense) in this part of the brain. Obviously, a neurophysiologist could give you a much fuller causal account of how this type of memory is stored in this part of the brain.

Another type of causal account would help to shed light on the different types of memory. Cognitive neuropsychologists could give us an immense amount of detail about this, but let me share with you a slightly simpler, clinical understanding. We can think of three broad types of memory: episodic, semantic and procedural. *Procedural memory* is the sort of memory at work when I am driving my car. It is not that I actually think about putting my foot on the clutch and changing gear as I approach a roundabout, but clearly I remember how to do this, because in fact I do it. Procedural memory is to do with 'knowing how' (and is associated with a part of the brain called the dorsolateral striatum), which is contrasted with declarative memory, which is to do with 'knowing what'. *Episodic memory* is the memory for episodes, for events in life. Remembering that Aunty Bertha was stung by a bee on the beach at Bognor would be an example of episodic memory. It can be split up further into *anterograde* and *retrograde* memory, where anterograde memory is to do with newly encountered information (in other words the sort of recall memory that I was speaking about before), whilst retrograde memory is memory for past events, such as the bee and Bertha in Bognor. And some conditions

---

7   Again, more details can be found in Hughes 2011b.

affect one type of episodic memory more than another. Finally, there is *semantic memory*, which involves memory for words and their meaning and also general knowledge. It is the store of our knowledge and the meaning of words. Although the event in Bognor with Bertha is tied to a particular time, my knowledge of bees is not episodic in this way. It is not linked to an episode that I can remember, it is just one of the things that I know. Semantic memory is said to depend on the *anterior* temporal lobe.[8]

Now there are further complexities. For instance, I have not mentioned working memory, which refers to the very short-term memory that allows us to retain information for just a few seconds and then disappears unless we use the memory. This is said to link to the dorsolateral prefrontal cortex. And clinical observation teaches us other things. For instance, most clinicians and many other people can recall someone they knew who had very distinct problems with memory and, perhaps, profound problems with speech and language, but who could none the less still play piano pieces perfectly from memory. So obviously this sort of procedural memory for music is stored somewhere else in the brain.

People also talk about emotional memory. This provides a coherent story of why the person who very quickly forgets events none the less seems to be affected in an emotional way by what is going on. For instance, the person trying to get out of the hospital ward, whose attempts to leave are constantly being thwarted, by the end of the day cannot remember all the particular episodes when he tried to leave, but he has nevertheless been left with a strong sense of frustration, which then erupts into some form of agitated and perhaps violent behaviour.

Now the point is that all of these causal explanations, in terms of different types of memory and different areas of the brain, can be very useful clinically in that we can understand the person's particular needs. One person may require written prompts for appointments, whereas someone else may require gentle verbal prompts to help them with their language problems, or the use

---

8   For a more detailed account of cognitive neuropsychology and the brain, see the excellent book by John Hodges (2007).

of pictures. In the case of the frustrated man trying to leave the ward, he requires an approach and the type of human encounter that will not leave him feeling just frustrated, but which might improve his well-being. Beyond clinical scenarios, these numerous different types of memory suggest that people can be engaged in numerous different ways. Here we might think, for instance, about the difference between recall and recognition.

The American neuropsychologist, Steve Sabat, talks about this in his book *The Experience of Alzheimer's Disease* (Sabat 2001). He makes the point that confronting someone with the requirement that they should remember three words will often lead to failure if the person has problems with recall. Nevertheless, if the words are then shown amongst other words, the person may well be able to recognize the words even though they cannot be recalled. A standard test of cognitive function involves asking people to remember the three words 'apple, table, penny'. In someone with Alzheimer's dementia of even a mild to moderate severity, they will quickly forget the three words. But if you say to them, 'Which of the following three words might have been one of the words you heard before?' and you give them words such as 'boat, sideboard, apple', people often recognize 'apple' as being a word they have just heard. One of the benefits of this is that it demonstrates the things that the person *can* do, rather than what the person *cannot* do.

Another phenomenon, often noted by relatives, is that the person with dementia forgets things in the recent past, but has a good memory for things in the distant past. They cannot recall yesterday, but can recall what their grandmother used to do before the war. This phenomenon was noted in 1881 by Théodule Ribot (1839–1916) and is known as Ribot's Law (even if the underlying cognitive mechanism is now in doubt).

The ability to remember things from long ago and the ability to recognize rather than recall suggest the potential importance of, for instance, museums or other cultural activities that draw upon the past (songs, say) as a way to engage with people with memory difficulties. Thus, in our own unit for people with severe dementia we have on loan a box of artefacts from the famous museum at

Beamish (www.beamish.org.uk), which helps to bring back memories and stimulate conversation and meaningful engagement amongst our patients.

Of course, there are caveats. Not everyone is typical. Some people will also have grave difficulties with speech, so that their understanding of things would have to be carefully negotiated rather than it be presupposed that they either did or did not understand and recollect. Communication would have to be adapted to meet the individual's needs. But meaningful activities remain meaningful because the person can still use certain bits of the brain, or certain pathways in the brain, in order to engage, understand, recognize and recall.

All in all, therefore, *causal* accounts of memory can take us a very long way. They tell us something about the person and how persons need to be understood and approached in a broad fashion. This is not a trivial point: understanding causal explanations helps us to understand how to help people with memory problems as individuals.

Constitutive accounts, normativity and the externality of mind

But there is more to be said about memory, which concerns our experience of memory. This is the constitutive account. It concerns the subjective experience of memory. What is this phenomenon of remembering? What is this phenomenological experience?

Now, one contention might be that our memories are private things that we have in our heads, which we are at liberty to share sometimes. There is obviously a sense in which this feels right, because even at this moment I could be remembering something that I am absolutely determined not to share with you. There is, however, an alternative theory of the mind, which suggests that this is unlikely to give us a proper account. This is the notion of the *externality* of mind.

According to this idea, we cannot have mental events without these events being constituted by worldly happenings. In philosophy there is the notion of *intentionality*, which is a technical term suggesting that there is a type of mental state that is always *about* something or *of* something. Thus, I cannot just have thoughts, I must have thoughts *about* such and such, where such and such will be (in some sense) in-the-world. Similarly, my memories are always memories *of* something. This feature of the mind is, according to externalism, quite general. In other words, all my thoughts, intentions, memories, hopes are peopled by the world. They inevitably involve the world and worldly things.

In discussing these matters I am obviously starting to open the lid on a whole can of philosophical worms that would need a good deal of attention. I am going to be a little cavalier about these worms, but let me just pick up one of them. This is to do with the notion of normativity.

Normativity is the idea that there are criteria of correctness, which allow me to say that the memory of Bertha-and-the-bee-at-Bognor was veridical: it really happened. The idea I want to use and emphasize is that intentional mental states – states of the mind which are inherently *about* or *of* things – must always display a type of normativity. If I intend to do something, there is something that must be the case for my intention to be the intention that it is. If I understand something, then certain things must follow. So if I say I understand what it means to 'add 2', then it must be that after '106' I will say '108'. We are normatively constrained, that is, we *must* do it this way if it is true that we understand what it is to 'add 2'. Now, of course, I can make things up and I can tell lies, but for the notion of understanding to be the notion that it is (for it to be the case that when I say I understand how to 'add 2' I do indeed add 2), for it to be possible for me to have memories in the same way that everyone else has memories (so that in a court of law my testimony means something), particular things in the world must be the case.

A major philosophical question is to do with the link between the mental things, in this case our thoughts and so on, and the world. How is this link achieved? How is normativity maintained?

Some philosophers argue that there is something like a platonic heaven in which these things are set down. They often talk of tracks along which things are constrained to move, but these tracks are not physical tracks. We cannot see them. They are akin to a non-physical type of love. Our platonic relationship happens somewhere in the heavens. So, too, the tracks that establish our normative responses are platonic. This, however, is a difficult position to defend.

Others talk in terms of *social constructionism* and suggest that the normativity is constructed by discourse and social interaction. In other words, we make up realities when we speak about them. It is in the nature of our discourse or talking that the normativity resides. Because we agree (at some level) to use language in this way, certain things are then true. A further development is a particular interpretation, derived from the philosophy of Wittgenstein, which suggests that normativity must be regarded as embedded in worldly human practices, namely the practices of remembering, intending, thinking, hoping and so forth.

I do not wish to try to pursue these philosophical ideas further here (but see Hughes 2011a). The point of the philosophy, however, is to emphasize again that remembering things is not just a matter of something happening inside the head, as it were behind the eyes. If some of the arguments I have been pointing towards have some validity, then the suggestion is that there is something quintessential about mental states such as memory, which means that they are at least potentially public and shareable. Even though they can be kept secret, if I *mean* or *think* something these must be things that could (at least potentially) be set out in public space for others to share. It is in their nature that this is true.

The mind is not in the head according to externalism (which I shall discuss further in Chapter 9) and, partly as a consequence – but also as a constitutive feature of such mental states – my memories must be essentially and at least potentially shareable.

Being persons in the world

Well, but what are the broader implications of this philosophizing? I would highlight two things. First, it means that a characterization of us *as persons* should involve the notion that we are situated in the world and this means being situated in cultures, histories, societies and so forth, as well as within our own particular skins with our own particular personal stories and so on. I would argue that the best characterization of us as persons is to say that we are situated embodied agents (Hughes 2001b, 2011a). Being situated, as a constitutive part of personhood, suggests that personhood is partly maintained by meaningful activities, by engaging with pictures, by using objects to reminisce, by making music and so forth.

The second thing I wish to highlight is the way in which, although we can be solitary, it is much more characteristic of us to have a form of being-in-the-world that is Being-with. This is to draw on some thoughts from Heidegger. He was interested in the nature of Being itself, or more specifically the nature of the Being of human beings. He talked of human beings as 'thrown' into the world, but not just as things, because for us other things have significance. We are decidedly not just things, because of the manner of our being which means that we inter-relate with the world and with others. The point is not just the ancient point that we are social animals, it is a little more than that, because the suggestion is that understanding the nature of our being *conceptually* points in the direction of our being-with-others.

Holding memories

So how do we hold memories? We hold them in public, in photographs, in pictures, in art, in cultural exchange, in historical archives, in museums and the like. And we do this not just as some form of add-on to real memory, which is neatly located in our heads, we do this because memories are *like this*: they are potentially and essentially public and shareable. But if this is the case, then in a situation where because of microscopic changes in particular parts of our brains memory is under threat, what better response than to try to engage the person in the broadest possible fields in which memories are held?

Many of us have lived through a quiet revolution when the asylums, with their back wards full of people with dementia, were shut down. People with longer-term conditions were, instead, housed in smaller institutions in the community. This is where many people with dementia are to be found today, sitting around the lounges of nursing and residential homes, often with very little stimulation except for the ubiquitous television, which they are mostly ignoring. Meanwhile, however, their needs as human beings – where a proper understanding of what it is to be a human person involves an understanding of the ways in which we are typically *situated* in our personal, family, cultural histories and in which, typically, our being-in-the-world involves being with others, not in a passive way, but in an engaged way – their real needs as human beings are as ignored as the television is by them. So the next revolution is to get people with dementia re-engaged with society, partly because this will do them some good therapeutically, but also because we cannot be the citizens of the world that we would like to be, in a moral and political sense, unless we have done all that we can to help our fellow citizens. Showing some sense of solidarity with older people, including older people with dementia, becomes a moral imperative once we see that our own standing as human beings-in-the-world is predicated on our ability to show solicitude for the Other.

CHAPTER 4

I Am Still the Same Person

Introduction

In the last chapter I spoke in passing of the notion of personhood – of what it is to be a person – and in this chapter I wish to enlarge upon my view of the person as a situated embodied agent. I have developed this idea before (Hughes 2001, 2011a), so do not wish to go over the philosophical roots of the situated embodied agent (or SEA) view of the person in any detail, but we have just uncovered some of these roots in Chapter 3. For if the mind is not just in the head and memories can be held by others, then the person must also be regarded as embedded in the context of the human world. We are, that is to say, all situated beings. But we are not just passive beings: we act in the world, we do things and we are agents. And finally we are also embodied. I shall say more about being embodied in the next chapter. In this chapter I shall consider personhood under three headings: in terms of, first, the challenge to personhood, second, the reply to the challenge and, finally, the implications of the reply.

The Nuffield Council Report

But before embarking, I just want to highlight the report *Dementia: Ethical Issues*, which was produced by the Nuffield Council on Bioethics (2009). I want to do this because the report set great store by the notion of personhood, which featured in the ethical framework it used to discuss ethical dilemmas (see Box 4.1).

Box 4.1 An ethical framework ─────────────────

Component 1: A 'case-based' approach to ethical decisions: In which each case is looked at individually, the facts are ascertained, ethical values are applied and the particular case is compared with other similar cases to identify similarities or differences.

Component 2: A belief about the nature of dementia: Dementia is regarded as a harmful brain disorder.

Component 3: A belief about quality of life with dementia: People with dementia can still live well if they are provided with the right care and support.

Component 4: The importance of promoting the interests both of the person with dementia and of those who care for them: These interests are in connection with both autonomy and well-being. Autonomy involves enabling and fostering relationships and supporting the person. Well-being includes both moment-to-moment experiences of contentment or pleasure, and more objective factors such as levels of cognitive functioning. The separate interests of carers must be recognized and promoted too.

Component 5: The requirement to act in accordance with solidarity: This implies the need to recognize the citizenship of people with dementia. We are mutually interdependent, so have responsibilities within families as well as in society as a whole.

Component 6: Recognizing personhood, identity and value: The person with dementia remains the same, equally valued, person throughout the course of their illness, regardless of the extent of the changes in their cognitive and other functions.

(Adapted from Nuffield Council on Bioethics 2009, p.21)

As can be seen, the sixth component of the framework is about recognizing personhood. Along with the fifth component, to do with solidarity, I think that our understanding of personhood underpins almost all of the other components in the framework. It is *persons* who have an interest in autonomy and well-being; the sense in which we are interested in quality of life is the sense in which this is important for *persons*; solidarity itself suggests our being-with-others as human *persons* in the world, and even the belief about the nature of dementia and the harm that it does (component 2 in the framework) reflects beliefs about human individuals, who are *persons*. Personhood is fundamental. Our thoughts about what it is to be a person are essential.

Challenges to personhood

It might be useful to start with a case example, such as that of Mr Bowes (Box 4.2).

Box 4.2 Mr Bowes

Mr Bowes was first diagnosed with dementia about 12 years ago. He was initially able to continue living with his wife in their family home. But after about three years he started leaving the house at odd times and his wife did not know where he had gone. He was becoming increasingly aggravated with her when she reprimanded him when he came home. He also started to show some problems with sleep. He was up pacing around the house for much of the night. His wife was becoming increasingly worn out. The situation was like this for about 18 months, but Mr Bowes then started to show some aggression towards his wife when she tried to reason with him. Finally he was admitted to a dementia assessment ward and from there it was decided he should move into long-term care. He became quite aggressive at times and needed to be given a variety of drugs to calm him down. Throughout this time his son and daughter and wife remained very involved. He always responded well to them when they visited, but he became more aggressive when they left. He was also persistently agitated during personal interventions, which were sadly becoming increasingly necessary because of incontinence. After a further couple of years, however, his physical strength and health declined. He became much easier for the home to manage; in the end he became immobile. He was transferred from his bed to a chair using a hoist. Once his language disappeared, he still clearly responded in various ways both to staff and to his family, who could tell whether he was sad or happy. But after a further year or so, he seemed to become quite indifferent to those around him. It was possible to catch his attention, but his responses were difficult to interpret. Now he mostly just stares into space, although he responds to noise, to voices and to touch, but not in a manner that allows meaningful communication. He is totally dependent on the staff for all of his needs. There is no evidence that he recognizes his family, who nevertheless continue to visit and to talk to him about family issues. Mr Bowes seems settled now, without his former agitation, but also without his previous abilities to communicate or to show meaningful reactions.

So what is the challenge to personhood? I think it comes in two guises. The first guise is the philosophical one. In its most shocking form, perhaps, it was put thus by Dan Brock:

> I believe that the severely demented, while of course remaining members of the human species, approach more closely the condition of animals than normal humans in their psychological capacities. In some respects the severely demented are even worse off than animals such as dogs and horses… The dementia that destroys memory in the severely demented destroys their psychological capacities to forge links across time that establish a sense of personal identity across time. Hence, they lack personhood. (Brock 1988)

Of course, there are some good philosophical arguments about the importance of memory and psychological continuity – from John Locke (1632–1704) to the contemporary Derek Parfit (1984), whose views we shall consider again in the next chapter – that support this view. In brief, people who are convinced by such arguments place considerable weight on the idea that memory is crucial to personal identity. Without memory, they argue, it is not possible for us to say that Mr Bowes is the same person now that he was when his dementia started 12 years ago. This is not the place to pursue these arguments (but see Hughes, Louw and Sabat 2006).

The challenge also comes in a second, everyday, guise. Husbands and wives of people with dementia say: this is not the woman or the man that I married. Rather than saying it is not a person *at all*, they suggest it is not *the same* person. This reflects, I think, the fact that dementia can be devastating. Recently, in our continuing care ward for people with severe dementia, a family carer told me that he still could not believe what had happened: he goes home and looks at photos of how his wife was just a couple of years ago and compares this to how she is now, when she is totally dependent and unable to speak.

A reply to the challenge

So, what is the reply to the challenge? I think the reply to the everyday challenge is, first, to be compassionate. It is often, after all, an emotional response requiring empathy rather than philosophy. But the answer I tend to give (if pressed) is to point out that we all change. I am very different, *as a person*, from the toddler that used to need to have its nappy changed; and very different, *as a person*, from the man who may also need to have his nappy changed in the future. The issue is complicated because what it means to be the *same* person is conceptually tricky. Again, the detailed discussion can be found elsewhere (see McMillan 2006). Suffice it to say that personal identity can be thought of in two senses. There is a quantitative sense: this computer is the selfsame computer that I was typing on last night. But perhaps it is not. Perhaps all of its component parts have been replaced overnight. It looks the same, but is actually quantitatively different: it is not the *same* one. Still, even if it is not quantitatively the same, in qualitative terms it is the same: it has all of the same qualities as the computer I left last night. So, too, I might be a different person in that I no longer look anything like the person that I once was (my properties have changed), yet I can still be identified as the same person because there are the qualities that contribute to my sameness: I may have ways of behaving that make me instantly recognizable. This may even be the case in severe dementia. But let us leave this debate to avoid its quagmires.

I think there is sometimes a simpler conceptual confusion in the everyday challenge to do with the difference between a change in personality and a change in personhood. My personality changes, perhaps, but precisely because it is *my* personality, my personhood (my standing as a person as such) is the same.

In a sense the answer to the philosophical challenge is easier. It is just to point out that we – as persons – are a lot more than mere linked memories. If to be a person you have to be able to remember what you did yesterday, then people with dementia are not persons. But to believe this is to indulge in the outlook of what the American ethicist, Stephen Post, called our 'hypercognitive society'. We put far too much emphasis on our cognitive abilities (being able to remember, calculate, verbally understand and the like). Reflecting on the work of Tom Kitwood from the Bradford Dementia Group, Post wrote: 'There is an emotional and relational reality in the lives of the deeply forgetful' (Post 2006, p.232). He continued: 'The person with dementia…is part of our common humanity as an emotional and relational being and therefore must be treated with care and respect.'

We can see in this statement the importance of solidarity, the fifth component of the Nuffield Council's ethical framework (see Box 4.1 previously). I share the view that being a person is more than just the ability to remember and thereby link up my mental states. I would, in addition, emphasize two things: we are embodied and we are situated.

There is an important sense in which to be me is to have my body. I shall discuss this further in the next chapter. But I am also situated in all sorts of ways that contribute to my being the person that I am. I am situated or located or embedded in my personal story or narrative, which links with the stories of others. I am situated in a cultural, historical, legal, social context and so on, with particular family relationships and shared experiences. All of these contexts still exist for Mr Bowes even in the midst of his severe dementia.

Implications

If this is, *at least in part*, what it is for me to be the person that I am, then it follows that, *at least in part*, what I am as a person can be held by others. My relationships, in a sense, sustain me. Even if I cannot remember, they can. And my bodily gestures are not *just* gestures perhaps: they may well carry contextual meaning and be reflections of my autonomy even if the rational expression of my autonomy is severely curtailed. As it says in the Nuffield Council report: 'The facts of bodily identity, and social connections, in particular, provide important grounds for considering a person as the same person throughout the full course of the illness' (Nuffield Council 2009, §2.50). The report went on to spell out some of the implications of this position; namely that:

> the views and values of the person before the onset of dementia may be relevant in making decisions;...the resources that the person has accumulated during their life may be used for their benefit; and that family and friends may retain responsibilities, and also expectations, that are normally assumed.

The report was also clear on the practical implications of the view that the individual with dementia was not a person at all, which are as follows:

> that the individual with severe dementia should not enjoy the protections of the law that are given to 'persons'; [and] does not have any interests, or none beyond those of other (non-human) living creatures; that those close to the individual...no longer have any interests or duties towards them; and perhaps that the views and values of the individual before the onset of dementia are no longer relevant in making decisions about their care. (§ 2.52)

It is because the person is still a person that we must encourage and enable them to make decisions, insofar as they are able; in other words, the broader view of personhood, which emphasizes the extent to which people with dementia can still value things, underpins much of the Mental Capacity Act in England and Wales and the Adults with Incapacity Act in Scotland. I shall enlarge upon the connections between personhood and decision-making capacity later in this book. But what we see here, by way of implications, is a moral imperative. It is a moral imperative to care because, at a deep level, we are inherently, mutually dependent, interconnected, human beings. This hearkens back to the philosophical line of thought that could be derived from Heidegger and Wittgenstein to which I referred in the previous chapter.

It is not, however, just that we can move from philosophical thought to what we should do or be; it is also that our experience of the world shapes our understanding of it. It is also that we see concrete manifestations of care – the daily visits of the husband or wife to see their spouse (such as Mr Bowes) in the care home, the sensitive handling by the care staff of the bedbound patient, the attention to his or her dignity, the formal reviews that seek to protect the human rights of the individual – we see concrete manifestations of care that only really make sense, to my mind, if we are dealing with persons: human beings with rights and interests, whose lives have value not solely because of what they may or may not be now, but also because of their relationships and histories, and because of the meaning that their lives have in this context.

Mr Bowes, for instance, is still the father of his children. He can no longer fulfil that role in the way that he once did when they were young, but the status of fatherhood cannot be taken away from him. It is because of this that they come to see him. They talk to him as a father, not as a stranger. They are situated in a context with him, which means that they cannot ignore his presence in the way that you can ignore other things in the world. It may be helpful to pursue this point. Clearly he is not like some physical object in the world that they could simply walk past and ignore. Alternatively, if he were just an animal, perhaps in the manner that Brock was describing, it would be difficult for them as human beings to ignore his presence. It is difficult to ignore animals that are in trouble. But their standing with respect to their father is more than this. It is at least like their standing to him as a fellow human being, but it is more than this too. And this is because of their shared history or narrative. Their stories involve his story at the level of biology (shared genetics), at the level of psychology (shared reactions) and at the level of their social worlds (shared experiences). There may also be shared spiritual experiences stemming from shared religious beliefs.

What if, however, the children of Mr Bowes were not devoted to him as they are? Say they are estranged because of the strict and uncompromising way in which he brought them up. Say, moreover, that his wife has died, so that there is in fact no one with whom his history or narrative can be shared. This would be extremely sad, but I do not think it would mean that Mr Bowes was not a person. Whatever happens, he is still situated, not just as an object, not just as a living thing, not just as any old human being, but also as this human being now. He will have relationships of some sort, with the carers who attend to him. They maintain his personhood and, true, they can do this well or badly. They can, indeed, strip him of all dignity and abuse him. But he is still, as this situated embodied agent, a person. And, I would argue, their standing in relationship to him precisely as a human being means that they have some obligations to sustain his personhood. These obligations stem from the shared nature of our moral world. Whatever our particular moral views, only an amoral world would allow us, not just to ignore our fellow human beings in trouble (because of course we can do that), but to deny that they have any call upon us; that is, to deny that we are situated in the world with them *as* human beings. It would not just be bad (immoral), it would be amoral because it would require that we did not see (conceptually) the other person as like us in this fundamental sense of being human.

Conclusion

It is easy to see why questions are sometimes raised about personhood in the context of dementia. This is both for everyday reasons, because we change drastically sometimes, and for deeper philosophical reasons to do with the nature of personal identity and selfhood. But the reply should be clear: if our view of personhood is the broad SEA view, then personhood persists in dementia as it does in other conditions. It partly persists, as we shall see in Chapter 5, through our bodies, as it does through our agentive acts. But we are not just bodies and our actions are not simply those of animals or artefacts; we are situated. That is, we are embedded in our world – the human world – where things inevitably have a significance. They have a human significance – a significance for us – even when the meaning, of a grimace or gesture, is not entirely clear.

The ethical implications of this are considerable. Our situatedness in the world as beings of this sort means that we cannot ignore things. Or at least, if we do, we are ignoring something of human significance so that our own standing as human beings is placed in a degree of jeopardy. I do not mean that every time we ignore a gesture or grimace, or a plea for attention, we stop being human. In fact, our standing as human beings is non-negotiable. But rather, we are not able to claim that we are leading our lives – being human beings – to the fullest extent possible. So we do place our own humanity in jeopardy. If a callous attitude towards suffering or requests for help were to become second nature – our way of being (or *modus vivendi*) – then talk of our inhumanity would start to make sense. So our situatedness as embodied and agentive human beings characterizes our personhood.

And personhood underscores, along with the other fundamental component of the Nuffield Council's framework – solidarity – our ethical dealings with the world of Others. Our situatedness and solidarity face us in the direction of the common good. In our encounters with people with dementia, therefore, it is in our nature to show concern and solicitude, not just as an emotional bodily reaction, but because this is who and what we are. The welcome new initiative of dementia-friendly communities (see footnote 4 in Chapter 2) is predicated on the demands of the common good. This relies on the community recognizing, in solidarity, the personhood of all its members, with or without dementia, and the inherent demand, thereby, for concern and solicitude. It should always have been thus. A broad view of personhood merely underpins, confirms and justifies the characteristics of a just and civilized society.

CHAPTER 5

The Body in Dementia

Introduction

The key text for this chapter comes from the French philosopher Maurice Merleau-Ponty (1908–1961): 'The body is our general medium for having a world' (Merleau-Ponty 1962, p.169). I want to show the relevance of this statement to dementia. But we must start again with clinical realities. So you should keep in mind the picture of Mr Bowes, whom we discussed in the previous chapter: a person with severe dementia, who is bed- or chair-bound, totally dependent for feeding, washing, toileting, and who is unable to communicate in an understandable way either verbally or non-verbally. But it is important to realize that Mr Bowes is not in some sort of persistent vegetative state. He is not comatose. He can be alert and he can interact with the environment, showing awareness of others and demonstrating a response to touch or to things that are said. But he cannot communicate meaningfully. In some people like Mr Bowes there may be obvious smiles or signs of displeasure. It can, however, be difficult even to interpret basic facial responses: is a grimace a sign of pleasure or pain? Again, perhaps, for the sake of realism, it is worth adding that carers (family, friends or professionals) who know him very well may be able to 'read' the signs of pleasure or displeasure more easily than other observers. It is this sort of person in the advanced stages of dementia that I wish to consider throughout this chapter.

But I want to add a proviso, which is that I do not think that Merleau-Ponty's thought and the arguments put forward in connection with this are *solely* relevant to people with severe dementia. They are relevant to people at other stages of dementia too. Let me expand on this briefly by harking back to the idea in Chapter 3 of the externality of mind. In that chapter, I drew upon the work of the philosophers Wittgenstein and Heidegger. In this chapter I shall use similar ideas derived from Merleau-Ponty. Towards the end of his book *Mind: Key Concepts in Philosophy*, Eric Matthews (2005) discusses the idea of solipsism. This is the idea that only one's own mind can be known to exist and, therefore, other minds and, indeed, the external world itself cannot be known for sure to exist. They may only exist in my mind, but not in reality. Again, thankfully, this is not an idea that needs to detain us. But in setting out Merleau-Ponty's argument against solipsism, namely that to have an idea of what it is to be alone entails having an idea of what it is not to be alone, Matthews says, 'our mental life is not to be equated with some *purely* 'inner' world: our minds are part of the public, social world' (2005, p.113). The phenomenal experience of being-in-the-world, for Merleau-Ponty no less than for Heidegger, is an experience of being-with-others. But Merleau-Ponty's spin on this was his emphasis on the importance of our bodily being-in-the-world. His work is sometimes summed up using the expression the 'body-subject'. This is to convey both that our bodies are minded, that is, they contain a subjective, personal viewpoint, and that our subjectivity (our mindedness) is embodied, that is, it does not float free in the ether, but is effective in the world through its bodily manifestations.

This account of what it is to have a mind, namely that it entails public or social engagement, can be seen at work very directly in the hands of the social constructionists, whom I also mentioned in Chapter 3. We find social constructionist thought being applied very directly to dementia in, for instance, the work of Steve Sabat (2001). He has convincingly shown, in a group of moderate to severely affected individuals (even if none was bedbound or quite in the situation of Mr Bowes), how the person's experience of selfhood is directly affected by the psychosocial environment, which can be malignant or benign. Their mindedness was apparent in public space, not least in the conversations that Steve was able to hold with them, even when they were starting to show some quite marked speech difficulties. So we should not forget that the 'body-subject', along with the implications that flow from this way of thinking of people, is relevant to people with less severe forms of dementia too. None the less, I have seen the greatest use for it in connection with thinking about severe dementia in people who cannot communicate their needs or wishes in a meaningful manner.

In the rest of this chapter I shall use the work of various philosophers or workers in the field of dementia to reflect on the significance of the body.

Merleau-Ponty

The idea I shall use from Merleau-Ponty is the one that I have referred to, that of the 'body-subject'. However, I recall from a conversation with Eric Matthews some years ago that this was not a phrase that Merleau-Ponty actually used. Still, the idea represents a breaking down of the distinction, which is usually most strongly associated with the work of René Descartes (1596–1650), between the inner and the outer. Even at this level of understanding, therefore, the notion of the body-subject is relevant to dementia because it starts to focus our attention on the importance of the person's body as a phenomenal experience.

This is how Matthews draws out some of the implications of the notion of the body-subject:

> as soon as we recognize that the subject of experience is a 'body-subject', whose being is essentially *in* the world experienced, then the objects of our perception cease to be simply objects that causally affect our sense organs and constitute instead the 'field' in which we move about and act and to which we respond. The 'meanings' that we find in the world are no longer…the simple result of causal processes… Instead, they become part of a reciprocal relationship in which the human body becomes the expression of a certain way of being-in-the-world. (Matthews 2002, p.59)

Through our bodies, therefore, we establish meaning in the world, not on account of causal processes but through our (meaningful) relationships. The implications of this for our thinking about dementia should be obvious: there is the possibility of meaning-making through our encounters as body-subjects, as creatures of this kind in-the-world.

But I want to look in a little more detail at what Merleau-Ponty says in *Phenomenology of Perception* about habit (Merleau-Ponty 1962). He discusses various things that we can do by habit: for example dancing, driving, making music or typing. He considers that these habits are neither a form of knowledge, nor simply involuntary actions. Instead, he says of typing: 'It is knowledge in the hands, which is forthcoming only when bodily effort is made, and cannot be formulated in detachment from that effort' (Merleau-Ponty 1962, p.166). He goes on to say: 'it is the body which "understands" in the acquisition of habit' (p.167).

Now, of course, this would make no sense if the body were thought of solely as an object in physical space. Instead, as a body-subject, the body can understand and create meaning. Merleau-Ponty is particularly keen on the example of music, where he discusses how an organist, presented with a new organ on which there is limited time to rehearse before a performance, can none the less create a world of affect, of emotion and of expression.

> Between the musical essence of the piece as it is shown in the score and the notes that actually sound round the organ, so direct a relation is established that the organist's body and his instrument are merely the medium of this relationship. (1962, p.168)

Merleau-Ponty describes the movements of the organist during the rehearsal as 'consecratory gestures': 'they draw affective vectors, discover emotional sources, and create a space of expressiveness...' (p.168). He concludes: 'Now the body is essentially an expressive space' (p.169). And it is shortly afterwards that he states: 'The body is our general medium for having a world' (p.169).

From this I wish to draw three points. First, we see the possibility that the body itself acquires habits and in doing so 'understands'.

The organist is not *thinking* that at this point he or she must play a series of rapid arpeggios with his or her hands whilst moving from the tonic to the dominant in a series of steps with the pedals. It just happens because the organist's hands and feet have been trained to acquire this capacity as a type of habit: these notes on the page elicit this response unmediated by any particular thought. (Indeed, musicians and other performing artists sometimes describe having quite random and disconnected thoughts whilst performing, for instance about the odd attire of the person sitting in row three.) At any event, the *body* 'understands', conveys meaning and so forth, at least insofar as it is a body-subject.

Second, the movements of the body, its gestures, are 'consecratory', which implies they are devotional or sacred in some sense; and the sense seems to be that they create affective, emotional and expressive space. One would really need to look back to and comprehend the French to understand Merleau-Ponty's meaning here. But let me just say that the use of the word 'consecratory', which seems particularly apt in connection with organ music, suggests to me the ultimately mysterious way in which *meaning* is created by music. It is, of course, tantalizingly difficult to pin down what the meaning of any particular piece of music might be; indeed, trying to pin it down in words seems likely to be entirely the wrong thing to do (at least if we think we can do this in any meaningfully *complete* manner). But we do gain here a sense of the body creating subjectivity – affect, emotion, expressiveness – not as something other than the body (it is not transcendental, albeit that music might sometimes also seem to point beyond the physical realm), but as a manifestation of its particular way of being-in-the-world as a body-subject.

Third, to return to the main text, 'The body is our general medium for having a world', we cannot, in any meaningful sense, be-in-the-world except through our bodies. But, in saying this, I take it that we are not simply saying that we need our bodies, as it were, instrumentally, to do the feeling and seeing and hearing, but also – if what I have been discussing above makes sense – our bodies provide us with the possibility of meaning, thought, intention, understanding. The difference is that between a highly 'intelligent' robot, which can navigate its way around an environment and pass comment upon it and even respond to simple comments and commands, and the human being who can 'draw affective vectors, discover emotional sources, and create a space of expressiveness…' (Merleau-Ponty 1962, p.168).

Well, let me spell out the relevance of these three points for thinking about dementia. First, perhaps, even in severe dementia, my body – as a body-subject – can still understand things. Second, perhaps my movements, gestures, grimaces must be taken seriously, even if I have severe dementia, because they are meaningful simply as human movements, gestures and grimaces. Third, it is through my body that I have the world that I do. And its meaning is not just a matter of knowledge and cognitive function, rather my human body, as a body-subject, also creates an affective, emotional and expressive space.

With a slight jump we could find ourselves speaking the language of Martin Buber (1878–1965), who emphasized the importance of *I–Thou* as opposed solely to *I–It* relationships. The Other – the human being with whom we are in relationship – is not just an object, an *It*, but is always a person of significance, a *Thou*. This distinction, in turn, became very important as an underpinning to person-centred care for people with dementia as advocated by Tom Kitwood (1997), which has had a very significant effect on the practice of dementia care over the last 20 years. So a line of thought can be traced from philosophy to practice, and its effects are to widen our conception of the nature of the human being and thereby to heighten our sense of the mutual concern we should feel for one another.

Eric Matthews

Professor Matthews is one of the acknowledged English-speaking authorities on the work of French twentieth century philosophers and a particular expert on the work of Merleau-Ponty. It is interesting, then, that his writings have often been relevant to dementia. If, for instance, given the notion of the body-subject, our mental lives are inherently part of the public, social world, albeit intimately connected with our brains, then our mental disorders can similarly be thought of as essentially public and social. 'Mental disorder is, in this sense, a disordered way of relating to the world, in particular to the human world: a disordered way of being-in-the-world, to use Heidegger's and Merleau-Ponty's expression' (Matthews 2007, p.101). In saying this Matthews is clear that, 'our personhood, our manner of being-in-the-world, is rooted in our biological character' (p.103). He continues:

> Personhood thus reflects biology: but conversely…our biological workings are, in part at least, those of persons: the ways in which we pursue even our animal desires, or express even our basic emotions, are conditioned by the human and social context in which we pursue them.

The broader view of personhood that emerges from these thoughts is of significance for our thinking about the person with dementia. In 'Dementia and the Identity of the Person' (2006), Matthews set out very clearly the arguments of John Locke and Derek Parfit concerning what it is to be a person, or (to be precise) to be the same person over time.

You will recall from Chapter 4 that John Locke, in the seventeenth century, and the contemporary philosopher, Derek Parfit, both hold that personal identity is a matter of memory or of what Parfit calls 'psychological continuity' and 'connectedness'. Thus, I am the same person today as yesterday because I am tied by consciousness, in particular by memory, to the events of yesterday. I am the same person today as yesterday tying my shoe laces up because I can recall tying them up on both days. This psychological continuity and connectedness amounts, in Parfit's view, to my being the same person. Or, as Locke famously said, the person is:

> a thinking intelligent being, that has reason and reflection, and can consider itself as itself, the same thinking thing, in different times and places; which it does only by that consciousness which is inseparable from thinking, and…essential to it. (Locke 1964, p.211; first published 1690, II. xxvii. 9)

Interestingly, when Locke talks of 'a man' as opposed to 'a person' he seems to take a broader view, which brings in the body:

> For I presume it is not the idea of a thinking or rational being alone that makes the idea of a man in most people's sense, but of a body, so and so shaped, joined to it; and if that be the idea of a man, the same successive body not shifted all at once must, as well as the same immaterial spirit, go to the making of the same man. (Locke 1964, p.211; 1690, II. xxvii. 8)

I have discussed this in more detail elsewhere (Hughes 2011, p.35). But it is clear that, as far as the term 'person' goes, according to Locke, for me to be the same person requires that I have memory. And this is, of course, a threat to the personhood of people with dementia who are losing their ability to recall yesterday or to connect psychologically with the person from yesterday. Matthews ultimately rejects the Locke–Parfit account:

> In one sense, Locke and Parfit are right: the possibility of forming a more complex sense of our own identity by thought and reflection is central to our concept of what a human person is. Where they go wrong is in ignoring the many other features of our concept of a person which form the background to this self-conscious life and which are important to the ways in which we treat persons. The other side to the notion of body-subject is equally important: not only does our existence as a person emerge from our embodiment, but also our bodily existence has to be understood as the expression of our individuality – at all levels – not just in the sophisticated communication of language and consciously recalled experience, but also even in such simple things as our body-language, our habits of behaviour, our characteristic mannerisms and gestures, and so forth. (Matthews 2006, p.174)

So the notion of the body-subject helps to sustain a richer view of what it is to be a person with dementia, even into the severer stages when mannerisms and gestures may be the main ways in which the person can engage with others. Towards the end of the chapter Matthews reflects on an acquaintance who, despite dementia, hangs on to her social graces and politeness. He comments:

Some core elements of identity as the person they have been continue to exist… This is not only because, except in the most severe cases, they retain some elements of their conscious identity in a way that a child necessarily cannot; but also because there survives something of their adult individuality in the habits of behaviour in which it has become 'sedimented' in the course of their development to adulthood and beyond. These characteristic gestures and ways of doing things are what keep alive the sense of the individual they once were, even if the more sophisticated levels of that individuality have been removed. (Matthews 2006, p.176)

Pia Kontos

Kontos is a social psychologist and associate professor at the University of Toronto. In 2004, she wrote an article entitled 'Ethnographic Reflections on Selfhood, Embodiment and Alzheimer's Disease', in which, in discussing Merleau-Ponty, she emphasized the way in which meaning emerges in social contexts:

words do not do their work by arousing representations associated with them. Language has inner content but the meaning of words is not entirely contained in the words themselves; rather, their meaning emerges from and is influenced by the contextual discourse. During interactions, words assume a gestural significance… (Kontos 2004, p. 840)

She has developed a notion of 'embodied selfhood', which derives from her reading of Merleau-Ponty, but also from Pierre Bourdieu (1930–2002). Bourdieu used the notion of *habitus*, which 'consists in dispositions, schemata, forms of know-how and competence, all of which function below the threshold of consciousness, enacted at a prereflective level' (Kontos 2006, p.207). Kontos feels that Bourdieu 'addresses the sociocultural sources of bodily practices' in a way that complements Merleau-Ponty. Hence, Kontos suggests that:

past experiences persist in the body in the form of transposable dispositions that collectively function as a matrix of perceptions and actions. They are embodied in the sense that the memory of them is not confined to the brain but is actually encoded in the muscles, nerves, and sinews of the body. (Kontos 2006, p.209)

This is the sort of 'sedimentation' to which Eric Matthews also referred. The idea is that some of our reactions will reflect experience and values that have settled in our being, not consciously, but in a pre-reflective manner so that our bodies react instinctively and yet with meaning.

Kontos's notion of 'embodied selfhood' is reminiscent of the characterization of the person as a situated embodied agent – the SEA view – described in Chapter 4. She describes 'embodied selfhood' as referring

> to the complex inter-relationship between primordial and social characteristics of the body, all of which reside below the threshold of cognition, are grounded in the pre-reflective level of experience, and are manifest primarily in corporeal ways. (Kontos 2004, p.837)

A similar thought is to be found in the work of Charles Taylor, who was also keen to establish the ways in which the world has significance for us and, moreover, the ways in which our bodies are minded in that they contain knowledge and understanding:

> Our body is not just the executant of the goals we frame... Our understanding is itself embodied. That is, our bodily know-how, and the way we act and move, can encode components of our understanding of self and world... My sense of myself, of the footing I am on with others, is in large part also embodied. (Taylor 1995, pp.170–1)

An idea that emerges strongly from this line of thought is that of 'tacit knowledge', to which I shall return in Chapter 10. This can be regarded as knowledge that cannot be made explicit but which is often associated with action: I simply do things without being able to say how (see Thornton 2013). We can see this idea as implicit in Matthews writing the following:

> Treating our body as part of our subjectivity...implies that not all aspects of our subjectivity – not all ways, for instance, in which

we may be purposive – need necessarily be fully 'conscious' in the sense of being objects of *explicit* awareness. For our bodies may have a purposive relationship to objects even if we do not cherish any *explicit* intentions for those objects. Reflex or instinctual actions, for instance, may be purposive but not consciously so... (Matthews 1996, p.92, emphases added)

If we now return to think of the person with severe dementia, such as Mr Bowes, who becomes agitated and aggressive during personal interventions, we can argue, along the lines of Steve Sabat (2001), that this man's behaviour is clearly still to be regarded as meaningful. His actions are agentive inasmuch as they are situated in a human context. They have, to use Kontos's memorable phrase, a 'gestural significance'.

Wim Dekkers

Similar lines of thought can be seen, too, in the work of Wim Dekkers, a physician and philosopher based in the University Medical Centre Nijmegen. In a book published in 2004 about palliative care and dementia, Dekkers discussed the person with severe dementia who is pulling at tubes inserted to feed him or her. The question is, do we disregard these gestures as signifying nothing but instinctual actions of no meaning, or do we give them some credence as in some way expressing the will of the person not to be interfered with? Again drawing on the work of Merleau-Ponty, Dekkers uses the notion of 'bodily autonomy' to argue that the human body lives its own life, that, 'The lived body demonstrates a "tacit knowledge"' (Dekkers 2004, p.125).

In a later chapter in the book *Supportive Care for the Person with Dementia* (Dekkers 2010), Dekkers re-used some of the material from the earlier work, but injected new thoughts. In particular, he was clearly impressed by the possibility of the 'sedimentation' of life habits that may influence actions even in severe dementia. Here is what Matthews had said in his chapter on dementia and personal identity:

we cannot say that a person ceases to exist as such once recall of their personal memories and the connected sense of who they are have been lost, as is presumed in (at any rate) the most severe cases of dementia. Something of their individuality survives even so. For on Merleau-Ponty's view a great deal more that is crucial to personal identity still remains in such a case. For us who care for them, all those elements in them that are not conscious or explicit will still remain the same. This will include anything that is due to genetic influences, as well as (probably more importantly) all that may originally have been conscious and reflective but has become 'sedimented' into habits. (Matthews 2006, pp.174–5)

In a similar vein, Dekkers wrote the following:

Cognitive capabilities of persons with severe dementia gradually disappear until the moment they are no longer capable of exercising their autonomy by making explicit decisions. This does not mean, however, that their bodily knowledge, which has been developed in the course of their lives, necessarily also disappears. Tacit bodily knowledge is based on the sedimentation of life narratives. Although automatisms get gradually lost, persons with severe dementia still have routine actions stored in their body. Behavioural patterns of persons with severe dementia may be interpreted as a remainder of what once has been 'real', that is, rational autonomy. They have nothing else at their disposal than these bodily movements. Although the body in severe dementia increasingly shows dysfunctions, it still remains a lived body and a body in which previous forms of autonomy have been inscribed. (Dekkers 2010, p.258)

Hence, according to Dekkers, we must take the person's bodily defensive movements seriously; they have 'gestural significance' (to quote Kontos again). This in turn takes us on to consider the practical upshot of much of this theorizing. Dekkers was concerned about the patient, like Mr Bowes, who has severe dementia where the attending physicians think it might be useful or beneficial to insert feeding tubes, either through the nose (using a naso-gastric tube) or through the abdominal wall into the stomach (using a percutaneous endoscopic gastrostomy or PEG tube).

It is not unusual in both of these circumstances for the person with dementia to try to remove the tube. In which case, he or she might need to be physically restrained if the tube is to be kept in place. But all of this could be very wrong if the person's attempts to remove the tube are, in fact, meaningful. 'If the argument of the lived body possessing tacit knowledge makes sense…it must be weighed alongside other reasons for trying, or not trying, to prolong a life by inserting feeding tubes' (Dekkers 2004, p.128).

Practical effects

What we see, therefore, is that the philosophy of Merleau-Ponty is actually suggesting practical conclusions concerning how we treat people with dementia. As Matthews says, 'an adequate philosophical theory of personal identity, however abstract it may sound, can have very practical consequences for the ways in which we think about, feel about, and deal with people with dementia' (2006, p.177).

The implications of this philosophy are broader than just whether or not to use artificial nutrition and hydration in someone with severe dementia. They should affect aspects of the day-to-day care of people with dementia. Matthews mentions the ordinary care which must, of course, be given to people with dementia, but he comments that this is no more than the ordinary care we might show to a pet animal, in terms of keeping the creature clean, fed and watered. Over and above such basic care, however, we can:

> help to keep a person's sense of self, and so of self-respect, alive longer. In part, this means reinforcing any remaining elements of conscious self-identity by talking to the person about our past shared life with them and encouraging their own reminiscences. This is something, of course, that is widely recognized and already practised by good carers. But we can also help to preserve the less conscious elements in a person's identity… One way we can do this is by making their physical surroundings as familiar as possible, so retaining the physical links with their past, which help to support the sense of selfhood. We can try to make it possible for the person to stay in their own home, with appropriate care

of course, for as long as it is practically and economically feasible (we should even be prepared to take some risks in order to do this, since it is part of human dignity that a person should be allowed to live their own life even if some risk may be involved). And when it is no longer feasible, and the person needs to be cared for in an institutional setting, every effort should be made to humanize that setting by including pictures, ornaments, items of furniture, and so on from the person's own home. (Matthews 2006, p.176)

Once again, it is striking how philosophical thought leads us in the direction of practical acts and, moreover, acts of such basic humanity that we might think they would always be pursued. This is sadly not the case. Reminding staff of the person's life history, taking note of current actions as clues to the person's needs, suggesting how beneficial it might be to have reminders of the past to hand, these are the daily tasks for those who seek to improve the care of people with dementia.

Conclusion

'The body is our general medium for having a world' (Merleau-Ponty 1962, p.169). The persistence of the human body in the human context is enough to establish that persons with severe dementia require more than ordinary care. They require a type of extraordinary care, not only because of the complexity of their physical condition, but because of the complexity of their metaphysical standing as persons amongst persons. They are situated embodied agents who demonstrate bodily autonomy and embodied selfhood. Behind these thoughts lie the influence of Merleau-Ponty and a host of other thinkers. Perhaps what we should be struck by here is the way in which through our bodies we interconnect in social space where our affects, emotions and our expressiveness are 'consecrated'. The person with dementia cannot step out of his or her historical embedding. But nor can any of us. As Merleau-Ponty famously wrote in the Preface to *Phenomenology of Perception*: 'Because we are in the world, we are *condemned to meaning*, and we cannot do or say anything without its acquiring a name in history' (1962, p.xxii). The stories of people with severe dementia are full of meaning, which we may or may not share. But to ignore the possibility of doing so – to fail to see their actions as significant and to fail to see our own responses as potentially conveying meaning – would be to undermine our and their standing as situated human beings. It would destroy the solidarity that should characterize our caring and solicitude.

PART III

Capacity and Incapacity

CHAPTER 6

'Capacity'

What Is It and So What?

Introduction

In this chapter I shall use a case vignette to raise difficulties over the assessment of one type of capacity that routinely arises in clinical practice (the capacity to decide on whether or not to return home or to go into long-term care in the face of cognitive impairment), which is called residence capacity. But the real issue to be discussed concerns our conceptual understanding of the notion of 'capacity'. I shall characterize the notion of 'capacity' as an ability involving practical know-how: an ability to participate in the relevant and particular sphere of facts and value-laden acts of the human world. I shall then highlight some clinical and legal implications of this view of capacity. Of central importance is the need to take a broad view of 'capacity', from the situated perspective of the individual, paying attention to values as well as to facts.

As I shall make clear, I am not interested here in the legal *definition* of capacity. One way in which the legal definition is sharpened is by making the point that it is *decision-making* capacity. The intention in saying this is to place capacity, or the exercise of capacity, firmly (as it were) in the head. But we have already seen (in Chapter 3) that things 'in the head', when they are mental things, have a tendency to make their way out of the head! Our mental life is inherently shareable. So, too, I want to say in this chapter, is capacity.

Finally, by way of introduction, I draw on documents in this chapter which were produced before the Mental Capacity Act 2005 (MCA) came into being. It might be considered that these are now purely historical. But they are useful in that they make a point I wish to emphasize: despite the best intentions, there is a tendency for certain forms of capacity to be medicalized in fact (*de facto*) if not in the law (*de jure*).

Approaches to capacity assessment

Even if values are, *de facto*, naturally spoken of by those concerned with capacity assessments, it may be that the introduction of values into the consideration of capacity is just wrong. To understand this further it is important to grasp the different types of assessment. There are three.

First, assessment based on *status* suggests that because a person has a certain condition he or she inevitably lacks capacity. We might say, if we adopt a status approach, that all people with learning or intellectual disabilities inevitably lack capacity. But most people strongly object to the status approach. It would be demeaning and wrong to say that all people with learning disabilities, or all people with dementia, or all people over the age of 90, lack capacity. For one thing, we would need to specify the capacity. A person with dementia might lack the capacity to manage his finances, but might have the capacity to consent to be given the flu vaccination. For another, it is just wrong to lump individuals together in this way. Whilst he lacks capacity to manage his finances, another person with dementia may retain that capacity. So we do not like the status approach (although we should note that purely having the status of being under 18 is enough for society to say that you lack the capacity to vote!).

Second, there is the *outcome* approach to capacity assessment. This suggests that, to determine if someone has capacity, we should look to the outcome of whatever the particular decision might be. The MCA specifically rejects this approach. In fact, it states that the person is allowed to be unwise and we are not allowed, just because she has been unwise, to say she lacks capacity. Unwise people are allowed to make silly decisions. Nevertheless, health and social care professionals do not feel comfortable knowingly allowing people to make decisions that might be harmful to them. If someone is inclined to make a harmful decision, there is a strong tendency for professionals to judge that they cannot have the relevant capacity. If a person knowingly chooses to do something with bad consequences, it is natural on this view to think that he or she cannot be thinking clearly. But the outcome approach is also rejected in England and Wales, even though we see assessments being based on outcome all of the time (Emmett *et al.* 2013).

Third, there is the *functional* approach, which is the one supported by the MCA. This suggests that the person has capacity when it is possible to see the relevant mental functioning. Can the person, that is, demonstrate that they are performing the correct steps in making whatever the decision may be? As we shall see, to have capacity under the MCA means being able to understand, recall and weigh up the relevant information (as well as to be able to communicate a decision). Functionally, then, we need to be able to see the person performing these tasks in order to say that he or she has capacity.

So, to return to my main point, it may seem as if values only creep in if we are tempted by the outcome approach. If we stick to a functional approach, it might be said, then there is no place for values. We simply have to observe the functioning of the decision-making process. But my point is that this ignores something fundamental, namely that we are not just computational machines: our decisions are made against a backdrop of values and inevitably, for example when we are weighing things up as part of our decision-making, values creep in when we decide to do things.

Nevertheless, there is another sense in which it might be that the introduction of values into the consideration of capacity just will not work. It might still be said that decision-making capacity is only about the functioning of the mind in making the decision, whether or not values are in play and whatever the values. This could be stipulated: the assessment of decision-making capacity *as such* should be made in a value-neutral manner. Perhaps I value orthodox medical treatment, or perhaps I have always rather valued alternative complementary therapies. The assessor of my capacity, it could be argued, has nothing to say about these values, he or she must solely have regard to the fact that I *have* weighed things up, whatever my premises or conclusions. The stipulation, then, is that we should adopt a strictly functional approach to the assessment of capacity.

This argument, which reflects the thinking of the MCA, can certainly be made. Capacity, however, as a result is a very narrow concept. *Decision-making* remains a bigger issue in real terms. In reality, making decisions requires evaluations and emotional judgements and they require a volitional component. If we cannot call these aspects 'capacity' – because of the stipulation that capacity should be a narrowly defined concept – we must still have a name for the evaluative/emotional and volitional components of decision-making.

Elsewhere, we have called these components competencies (Hughes and Heginbotham 2013). Hence, we have three things: cognitive capacity (the legal, functional aspect of decision-making, which mainly involves our cognitive or higher mental abilities), evaluative competence and volitional competence. Evaluative competence 'is the ability to make sense of the available cognitive information in the context of beliefs, values, and life choices. Evaluation is inherently social and/or emotional and may be guided by both conscious and unconscious factors' (Hughes and Heginbotham 2013, p.756). Volitional competence 'is the ability of the person to generate actions from a set of facts, beliefs, and desires. At its simplest it means agreeing that the decisions taken cognitively, subject to some evaluative assessment, should be enacted' (p.756).

The point of all of this is that we should think very broadly when we are making decisions for other people and when we are making judgements about their abilities to make decisions. We are not just cognitive computational machines. We are, amongst other things, emotional, evaluative and volitional creatures too; and our decision-making reflects our complex make-up. Judgements about the decision-making of others must allow enough space for this breadth of consideration.

So far, and in the rest of this chapter, I have been considering the MCA, because I work in the jurisdiction in which this law applies. Other countries have other laws. None the less, the conceptual and ethical issues being raised here will apply to all countries where the human rights of citizens, whether or not they have dementia, are taken seriously. In this chapter I consider the question 'What is "capacity"?' Our conceptual understanding of 'capacity' has implications for clinical practice and for the law. In a somewhat subversive way, philosophical discussion often serves to complicate matters, but it seems entirely appropriate to raise some questions and to try to show the complicated connections the notion of capacity makes with other features of our lives.

I shall start with a fictional case vignette (Box 6.1), but one based on real material. A feature of this sort of practical philosophy is that it is not just a matter of philosophical analysis informing practice, but the realities of practice can influence the philosophical understanding as well: there is two-way traffic. So I shall use the vignette to raise the question 'What is 'capacity'?' and I shall then consider the practical implications of this for clinical practice and for the law.

Box 6.1 Mr Adams

Mr Adams is a 75-year-old widower who lives alone. His only son lives at the other end of the country and rarely sees his father. Mr Adams is admitted to the general medical ward from the casualty department having had a fall. His neighbours had heard the thud as he fell. Having been admitted, Mr Adams is found to have a chest infection. This is treated and he gradually improves. He was quite confused when he was admitted and, whilst this also improves, he seems to be left with a degree of memory impairment and disorientation. He frequently wanders off the ward and has to be reminded he is in hospital. The medical team arranges a brain scan and finds evidence of two, very small, discrete strokes. They make a diagnosis of mild to moderate vascular dementia. The social worker speaks to the neighbours, who say they have been worried about Mr Adams for some time because he wanders out in the evenings. The occupational therapist takes Mr Adams home on a preliminary visit and finds the place very messy, with old food in the cupboards, evidence of burnt pans and a large quantity of bank notes lying on the bedside table. Mr Adams is jolly and optimistic. He says he can manage with the help of his good neighbours and he makes plausible excuses for the things found to be awry in his home. He states very definitely his wish to go home. It is noted on the ward, however, that he seems sometimes to believe he is still in the army. The medical team present all this information to an old age psychiatrist and ask for help in deciding whether Mr Adams has the capacity to make a decision concerning his future care and whether or not he should go home.

Who decides on Mr Adams's capacity to decide where to live?

Mr Adams's story is common enough. It is interesting to notice, therefore, that the assessment of capacity in this sort of situation, which would be considered routine in the practice of old age medicine and psychiatry, was seemingly not regarded as routine by the Lord Chancellor's Department back in April 2002. At that time, the Lord Chancellor issued leaflets intended to provide help and guidance around decision-making (Lord Chancellor's Department 2003), which stated:

> The *only* decisions which health professionals can make on behalf of people unable to make their own decisions relate to health care and treatment. They have *no authority* to make any other sorts of decisions, such as personal or welfare decisions. However, health professionals *may* have a role to play, in conjunction with relatives, carers and social care agencies to protect vulnerable people from abuse or exploitation. (emphases added)

From this it would appear that the doctors and occupational therapists looking after Mr Adams have 'no authority' to make decisions about his going home, inasmuch as these are 'personal or welfare decisions'. It might be objected, of course, that there is sometimes little or no clear water between, on the one hand, healthcare decisions and, on the other, personal or welfare decisions. It is relevant to note that, under the present Mental Health Act (1983), a ground for detaining someone with a mental disorder is the risk that the person's health will deteriorate. In the present case, it might be that Mr Adams's health will deteriorate if he lives alone (if, for instance, he cannot be persuaded to accept extra support). Yet, according to the Lord Chancellor's leaflets, the decision to remain living on his own is not a medical one. The ambiguity arises because the notions of healthcare and personal welfare are not conceptually distinct. This ambiguity cuts both ways: not only do medical considerations become relevant in all sorts of personal decisions, but also, even in the seemingly straightforward case of treatment decisions, there will be relevant social and personal concerns.

Deciding where a person should live is referred to as a 'more complex' decision, which will need to be made in conjunction with family, appointed decision-makers and other members of the care team. Ultimately such decisions may have to be made by the court. The Lord Chancellor's leaflets explicitly state, in connection with decisions about where a person should live, that 'The people who care for you have no right to force any major decisions on you if it is clear that you object.'

We find ourselves, therefore, in deep water. What might seem like a routine decision in medical practice – involving a decision concerning capacity – turns out to be far from straightforward. If in the case of Mr Adams it is decided that he does not have capacity to decide where he should live in the future in the face of his clear statement that he wishes to go home the matter could, perhaps, be referred to the court. Yet, actually, decisions like this *are* being made daily by multidisciplinary health and social care teams without reference to the courts. Where there is *good* clinical practice, such decisions are being made on the basis of a broad consensus concerning the patient's best interests (which will take into account the views of all concerned, including the expressed views of the person him or herself and significant others). But the rights of the person without capacity are not formally protected in these routine decisions about future 'placement'.

Whatever one's views about Mr Adams, his case immediately stresses the importance of decisions about capacity. For, once a decision is made that someone lacks residence capacity, a whole train of events follow that might have profound consequences for the person concerned. He might find himself in an institution not of his choosing, in effect being deprived of his liberty and, thus, of a basic human right. So, huge matters hinge on the *routine* assessment of Mr Adams's capacity. If, *de jure*, the complex matter of residence capacity is one that needs considerable safeguarding, *de facto*, it is a routine medical decision (Emmett *et al.* 2013). And this should prompt us to take the question 'What is "capacity"?' seriously.

What sort of question?

Whilst it is important to answer the question 'What is "capacity"?', it is equally important to establish what sort of a question this is. I am not seeking a simple definition, nor is the question answered by reference to legal criteria, although it is as well to be aware of such criteria. The MCA, for the first time in law in England and Wales, defines capacity and sets out criteria by which incapacity should be judged. This is shown in Box 6.2.

The criteria in Box 6.2, however, do not address the issue I wish to consider, namely: *what is it for me as a person* to have or not to have a capacity? The point is that capacities link to what we are. In this sense, it is a metaphysical question: the question is about the nature of things, or more precisely, it is about what constitutes us as beings with or without these capabilities.

Seeing the relevance of the question when it is *this* sort of question should bring into mind something about the structure of clinical practice. It is underpinned by law and ethics.

Box 6.2 The definition of incapacity from the Mental Capacity Act 2005 (MCA)

A person lacks capacity in relation to a matter if at the material time he is unable to make a decision for himself in relation to the matter because of an impairment of, or a disturbance in the functioning of, the mind or brain. (MCA Section 2(1))

A person is 'unable to make a decision' if he is unable:

(a) to understand the information relevant to the decision,

(b) to retain that information,

(c) to use or weigh that information…, or

(d) to communicate his decision (whether by talking, using sign language or any other means). (MCA Section 3(1))

In fact, clinical practice is typically, at one and the same time, legal and ethical in nature. This has become more and more obvious to clinicians in recent years as various medical scandals have hit the headlines. But, as Figure 6.1 indicates, clinical practice also has philosophical underpinnings. As with law and ethics, philosophical issues are inherent to practice.

Acting in one way can imply certain philosophical stances; alternatively, the philosophical underpinnings might influence clinical decisions. This simply emphasizes the two-way nature of the traffic between practice and philosophy. In addition, it highlights the importance of philosophy, not solely for clinical practice, but for the ethical and legal aspects of practice too. Recognizing this suggests that our capacity legislation should reflect underlying intuitions concerning what it is to be a person with (or without) particular capacities.

Foundations of Clinical Practice

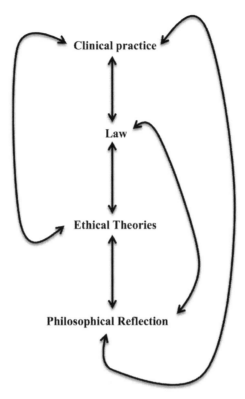

**Figure 6.1 The relationship of clinical practice
to law, ethics and philosophy**

So what is 'capacity'?

Definitions of capacity naturally invoke the notion of ability. This in turn suggests something practical: being able to do something. So my characterization of 'capacity' is that it involves practical know-how or knowledge. The idea of practical knowledge, or knowledge in acting, is an ancient one. Ethical decisions have, for instance, been conceived as a matter of practical knowledge, according to which our actions themselves involve and reflect knowledge relevant to the issue in question.

The notion of knowledge in 'practical knowledge' brings into play facts. There will, therefore, be facts that are relevant to whether or not Mr Adams has residence capacity. The notion of practice in 'practical knowledge' suggests actions or doing things. But more than that, 'practice' suggests the human world in which human practices are embedded.

To unpack this slightly, I do things in the world. What I do will, in some sense (at least potentially), have an effect on the world. Even an expressed opinion has this potential. For philosophical reasons the parenthetic 'at least potentially' needs to be in place to cover the possibility of someone acting on his or her own. The philosophical position I am reflecting would have it that, inasmuch as an action is one that makes sense to us as human beings (or has that potential), to this extent it must be one that conforms to normative standards of understandability. That is, even Robinson Crusoe (before the arrival of Man Friday), inasmuch as his actions are potentially understandable, must be acting in conformity with rules that govern human practices. There are norms of practice: ways in which practices either do or do not make sense to us *as* human practices, whether these are words or physical acts. These practices, however, which give sense to what we do, in order to perform the normative job required of them (i.e. in order to provide a non-negotiable sort of certainty to what we do), must be embedded in the world. They must be part of the fabric, the woof and warp, of our human world. So, not only does practical know-how bring in facts, it also brings into play the idea of agents acting in the world. For someone to have (or not to have) a capacity is for them to have (or not to have) the ability to participate in the relevant and particular sphere of facts and value-laden acts of the human world.

Now there are various philosophical positions that lend support to the thoughts I have been expressing. For instance, to return to the writings of Heidegger, in which the human existent is referred to as *Dasein*, we find the following: '"world" is not a way of characterizing those entities which Dasein essentially is not; it is rather a characteristic of Dasein itself...' (Heidegger 1962, p.64). This suggests that the human being is not to be thought of as standing separate from the world. He or she is part and parcel of the world and the world is involved in what it is for that person to be the person he or she is. Merleau-Ponty's notion of the 'body-subject', which we encountered in Chapter 5, makes the same point. Similarly, the situatedness of the SEA view (in Chapter 4) also stresses our embededness in the world, with all that this entails.

In summary, therefore, a capacity is an ability involving practical know-how: an ability to participate in the relevant and particular sphere of facts and value-laden acts of the human world. Inherently involved in the having or not having of a capacity, therefore, are particular facts, but also the person's situated nature as an embodied agent acting in the cultural, psychological, social, moral and spiritual world. In short, a capacity involves facts and values. But the values are as quintessential as the facts.

So what?

There are at least two broad areas of concern consequent upon the understanding of 'capacity' as involving both facts and values. First, there are implications for clinical assessment, second, there are implications for the law.

Clinical assessment

In deciding whether or not Mr Adams lacks capacity to make the required decision about going home, it becomes clear that we cannot simply have recourse to some putative objective fact. We also need to take into account Mr Adams's engagement with the world. Of relevance is his assertion that he has neighbours who can help him. It might be entirely true that his neighbours would be willing to continue to support him. If so, he has demonstrated a type of practical knowledge, showing that he has a grasp of his need for help and that he knows what action to take to manage. Equally, however, it might be that the neighbours are exhausted and cannot support him any longer. In which case, his belief that he can call on them shows a lack of understanding of the true situation. Still, it might be that their exhaustion needs to be brought to his attention in order for him to reconsider his position.

If he really cannot grasp their difficulties in continuing to provide him with support, he thereby shows that he lacks an element of the practical know-how that would allow us to say that he has capacity to make decisions about his future care. Coming into play here, therefore, are elements of his evaluative competence: his ability to judge emotionally and make evaluative judgements. But he needs to be informed of the other options, for instance that he might yet be able to live in the community with appropriate home care provided by social services.

Mr Adams is embodied, too, and there will certainly be factual matters that are relevant to whether or not he has capacity. So, for example, the finding of small strokes in his brain, linked to particular deficits in cognitive function, are facts that have to be taken into consideration. Similarly, the fact that he is otherwise fit is important. It means, on the one hand, that he can do things to look after himself, that he can take action to avoid harm, but, on the other hand, it means that he can wander at times and, if disoriented, this might itself place him in danger. Hence, we see elements of his volitional competence assuming importance in his ability to exercise his cognitive capacity.

Finally, Mr Adams is an agent, as shown by his practical and decision-making abilities. He continues to engage with his environment in a way that indicates his wishes and his needs and, within certain limits, he is able to manipulate things to satisfy those wishes and needs.

The points made previously might seem unremarkable. However, they are remarkable when it is considered that we are engaged in an assessment of Mr Adams's capacity to decide on whether or not he should go home or into long-term care. For the assessment of capacity is often presented as if it were simply a straightforward objective test.

There are three points to make. First, although there are some specific legal 'tests' for capacity and although clinicians have tried to devise appropriate measures of capacity (Vellinga *et al.* 2004), the earlier discussion illustrates the extent to which judgements about decision-making are inherently too broad to be pinned down by such tests or measures. Even in well-conducted research seeking to establish correlations between capacity and scores on cognitive tests, investigators have to make reference to what are inevitably subjective assessments of capacity.

Second, in the case of the decision as to whether or not to live independently or to accept long-term care, there are no accepted tests or assessments available upon which to judge capacity. The matter will remain one of judgement based upon uncertain probabilities. A tool could be developed, which might have the benefit of standardizing such assessments, but which could also exclude consideration of important elements of the person's situated agency (their lifelong tendency to solitude, for instance). In any case, at root, a new tool would be based on subjective assessments.

Third, the most crucial factor in the decision around Mr Adams's residence capacity in this respect will be the outcome of the occupational therapy home assessment. This stresses, again, the practical and volitional nature of decision-making. The same applies to an assessment of someone's capacity to manage their financial affairs: can the person actually handle everyday financial transactions? Similarly, in making a will, the person must demonstrate practical knowledge: the testator must understand the nature of the act of making a will. This is not just a piece of factual knowledge, it requires understanding of the world of relations, where people will have certain sorts of claims and where the act of making the will has consequences in the world.

These points make the broader consideration of capacity, as an ability to participate in the relevant and particular sphere of facts and value-laden acts in the human world, really remarkable. For one thing, what keeps on emerging is the importance of shared values that allow us to judge whether or not Mr Adams really has residence capacity. This follows from the situated nature of Mr Adams as an agent in the world. Judgements about his responses to the situation will depend on shared views about risk, on shared estimations concerning the importance of autonomy, on shared views over what is in Mr Adams's best interests, and so on. But assessing a person's capacity is often perceived as a straightforward matter of applying criteria or some form of test. This is decidedly not the case when the broader view is seen.

The upshot is that capacity is nothing like the 'clean' concept that it once might have seemed to be. The point of judgements concerning capacity, at least when it comes to treatment decisions, is that they should allow us to decide whether someone is able to give valid consent. Valid consent depends upon the person being informed, uncoerced and having capacity. In the absence of capacity we should move to consider acting in the person's best interests if his or her previous wishes are not appropriately recorded. In the clear-cut algorithm, capacity is objectively assessed and then, in its absence, best interests are pursued. In the muckier world of values, which I have been suggesting above, the assessment of capacity already involves the values of the patient. Mr Adams's wish to go home (which would feature in an assessment of his best interests) is not irrelevant to judgements about his decision-making abilities. The high priority he gives to his independence, a judgement concerning the importance of autonomy in comparison with the risks associated with wandering for Mr Adams, along with the occupational therapist's view that he could be adequately supported in the community, would all have a bearing on the judgements about his decision-making abilities concerning his long-term care. The distinction can be put in this way: either the assessment of capacity is an internal affair, with reference solely being made to the cognitive capacity criteria, or the assessment of capacity is externalist, with reference being made to outer, situational or contextual events. My characterization of capacity, as an ability involving practical know-how, suggests that the correct view is the broad one, where capacity assessments are recognized inherently to involve judgements of value concerning the situated embodied agent as well as factual matters involving cognitive functions.

Legislative concerns

The second area of concern, consequent upon the understanding of 'capacity' as involving both facts and values, centres on the implications for the law. The broad characterization of capacity implies that judgements about decision-making must inherently involve both facts and values. An ability to participate in the relevant and particular sphere of facts and value-laden acts in the human world will mean that assessments of capacity are not disconnected from issues relating to praxis. That is, decision-making will entail: first, the person being able to do something in the world; and, second, a judgement concerning the decision that recognizes its situated nature and is itself situated.

The concern becomes more acute when the notion of generic incapacity criteria is considered as an alternative to diagnostic criteria as the basis for involuntary psychiatric treatment. The broad characterization of 'capacity' that I have commended places an emphasis on the shared values implicit in this notion. But as Dickenson and Fulford comment:

> criteria which depend on *shared* values…are a recipe for the values of the majority being imposed on the minority. …the risks here will be especially large if the value judgements concerned are not recognized for what they are – if the generic incapacity criteria are thought to be objective scientific criteria and a matter solely for expert witnesses to determine. (Dickenson and Fulford 2000, p.88)

Later, citing Kennedy (1997), they suggest:

> bioethical (and legal) criteria of incapacity, or at any rate those criteria currently advocated, provide no way of distinguishing between someone who lacks the capacity for autonomous choice and someone whose choice is merely different from everyone else's. (Dickenson and Fulford 2000, p.160)

This is not to suggest that judgements concerning capacity cannot or should not be made. However, it points towards the complicated nature of those judgements, which will be inherently evaluative and located in the sphere of shared (and disputed) values. They will not simply be matters of fact allowing of objectively verifiable tests. Laws concerning incapacity must encourage broad interpretation based upon the perspective of individual persons as situated embodied agents, which should necessitate awareness of relevant facts, but also of the values inherent to human action.

Conclusion

The case of Mr Adams is routine in medical practice, but it shows the difficulty of deciding whether someone has capacity to make a decision concerning where he or she should live in the future in the face of cognitive impairment. This particular decision concerning residence capacity raises a problem concerning who decides, because – whilst it is reasonably regarded as a 'personal and welfare' matter – clinical considerations are important too. I have characterized 'capacity' as an ability involving practical know-how: an ability to participate in the relevant and particular sphere of facts and value-laden acts of the human world. This has clinical implications: capacity cannot solely be decided by reference to cognitive function tests. Decision-making will always involve subjective and evaluative judgements, which will need to take account of the situated, embodied nature of the person's agency. Judgements about decision-making will be inherently practical, rooted in the person's ability to participate in the relevant way in the world. Assessing capacity brings into play the mucky world of shared and disputed values. There are also legal implications: there is the worry that incapacity legislation will not prevent injustices. These will occur if society and the courts are too interested in putatively objective tests and minimizing risks. The need for a broad interpretation of decision-making – to involve cognitive capacity and, in addition, evaluative and volitional competencies from the situated perspective of the individual – will remain crucial.

It was a concern with the possibility that courts might be swayed more by objective tests than by individual (situated) abilities in judging the capacity (or competence) of a person with dementia that led Sabat to state: 'The means by which we evaluate, and arrive at our conclusions about, the afflicted person's competency may well ultimately be a test of our own competency as thoughtful, judicious, humane human beings' (Sabat 2001, p.334).

CHAPTER 7

Capacity Legislation in Practice

Balancing the Personal and the Polis

Introduction

The Mental Capacity Act 2005 (MCA) came fully into effect in England and Wales in October 2007. For those who work with people who cannot make decisions for themselves, the MCA was largely greeted with a sense of relief and it has, largely, been embraced as a welcome clarification of the law. Nevertheless it is not all plain sailing. In this chapter, using scenarios based on real cases but significantly anonymized, I want to point towards a tension that runs through the implementation of the MCA. In doing this, I think I am pointing to a tension which exists anywhere that the rights of those who cannot make decisions for themselves are a concern, especially when others wish to help. In other words, this is a tension for any civilized society.

The tension I refer to is not new: it is the tension between a tendency to paternalism on the part of doctors and the paternalism of the state when it interferes with professional judgements and relationships. It is also the tension between the personal therapeutic relationships between health and social care professionals and their clients or patients on the one hand and, on the other, the power and bureaucracy of the *polis*. This is the Greek word for city, but can be taken to imply the city-state. The question is to what extent should, or when should, the demands and strictures of the state interfere with the personal interactions involved in one-to-one everyday care. One way to put this would be to say that the tension is to do with where the line between ordinary and exceptional practice should be drawn. In the ordinary case, there is no warrant for the state to interfere. In the exceptional case, the public and the law might well be warranted in insisting that healthcare is closely regulated. There is no doubt that the MCA has shifted the line. In many ways this is a good thing (it should have improved practice), but from the shop floor it can sometimes seem as if the line has moved too far. This is what I wish to tease out in considering how the MCA has been put into practice: to what extent does the MCA impose unwarranted interference in professional, clinical judgements and decisions?

I want to add that the issue runs deep, for at root it is to do with the moral basis of health and social care practice: what is it to be a good clinician? What is it to be a good social worker? The tension over drawing the line stems (at least in part) from the worry that this is being gradually undermined in favour of a more bureaucratic (and legalistic) approach.

Ethical tensions and capacity

The sorts of tension I am referring to can be epitomized by the case of Mrs George (Box 7.1).

Box 7.1 Mrs George ─────────────────────────────

Mrs George had been refusing the visits of her home carers for some while. She also became aggressive with the district nurse who called to oversee her use of insulin injections for her diabetes. Because she had threatened the nurse with a stick it was judged unsafe for the nurses to visit. Hence, because of her marked forgetfulness, Mrs George was probably not receiving her insulin.

Mrs George had a good relationship with a carer who continued to visit to help her with her shopping. The initial question concerned her capacity to make decisions about her need for care. The question about her capacity is difficult, but if it is deemed she lacks capacity, the decision about her best interests is still difficult and full of moral uncertainty. Is it better to risk trying to support her at home, to allow her independence? Or are things so precarious that a hospital admission, which would seem very likely to be followed by longer-term institutionalization, should be forced upon her in her best interests? So, the first step is that she needs an assessment of her capacity.

An initial point to make is that there are different types of capacity to be assessed. There is the capacity to make a judgement about hospitalization and the capacity to make judgements about her treatment and about how her treatment should be monitored. There are two minor points to make. First, separating these capacities is not completely straightforward. Her potential hospitalization involves her treatment, but these things are not the same thing. There is a particular issue to do with the insulin, which is quite different from whether she is admitted to hospital. But, equally, what she has to eat is not totally separate from her diabetic control. The point is that the assessments require quite a bit of careful conceptual thought in order to be clear which capacities are being assessed and, therefore, what information is material to the decision in question. The second minor point follows: Mrs George might object to an interview that has to go over, in a rather pedantic way, whether she retains, understands and weighs up the material information with respect to each of these separate mental capacities. It might, indeed, be unrealistic to expect that she will go along with all of this.

Although I have called these points 'minor', actually it will be seen that they are of some consequence. They lead on to the major point I am pursuing. It might previously have been that a clinician would have made, in conjunction with others involved, including family, a global judgement about Mrs George's relevant capacities. Now, however, this is not legally safe. Grounds have to be given with respect to each separate capacity.

This is what the MCA would suggest, but without really any acknowledgement that the judgements about the capacities to be assessed can themselves be conceptually complex. Note, however, that the need for this level of legalistic detail has a direct impact on patient care. Understandable worries, perhaps, about paternalism have led to an insistence on more thorough assessment. But the upshot is that Mrs George becomes irritable with the questioning, which starts to feel like an interrogation and which tends only to point out problems with her decision-making. The concern is that potentially therapeutic relationships may be damaged in the process.

My point must not be misunderstood. Actually, it does seem absolutely appropriate for these sorts of assessment to be made carefully. The MCA has performed a useful function inasmuch as it has made this all clearer: it is better for all those who depend on others to make their decisions. But there is a potential downside, which becomes more prominent the more the inclination to pursue assessments in a slavishly bureaucratic way is encouraged. And what has to be admitted is that an immediate effect of the MCA has been a tendency (at least) to slavish bureaucracy, sometimes without proper attention to the priority of the therapeutic relationship.

It is this that undermines an alternative possibility, which is to see an ethical requirement that people with impaired decision-making capacities need good quality judgements made about them in ways that are helpful, that minimize distress, that are truly responsible (i.e. where the person making the judgements takes responsibility for them, which does not simplify to an insistence on filling in the right forms) and are made on the basis of considerable experience. Rather than 'paternalism' this has sometimes more sympathetically been called 'parentalism', which stresses the idea of nurture and concern in the face of real dependency.

> Parentalism has its roots in a phenomenon essential to being a human person, namely, that a human person does not spring into being fully formed as an independent agent but develops through psychosocial relations with human parents. Parentalism signals the essential interconnectedness of all human persons and is rooted in the basic response to the needy other that such relationships engender. (Agich 2003, p.48)

Box 7.2 Mr Jenkins

Mr Jenkins lives in a nursing home. He has suffered several small strokes. He remains mobile, but is frequently irritable and he tends not to comply with the help offered to him. He gradually becomes more and more withdrawn. Staff feel that he may well be depressed. He seems to be permanently low in mood. The general practitioner (GP) visits and prescribes an antidepressant tablet. But by this stage Mr Jenkins is starting to refuse his medication. He is also eating less. It is clear that he is deteriorating. The nurse in the home thinks that the medication should be given covertly; in other words it could be hidden in his food or drink. She speaks to the family, who agree because they are very worried about him. But this must be sanctioned by the GP.

The GP who prescribed the medication is on leave and the other doctors are unwilling to get involved, saying that they would prefer to await their colleague's opinion, because she knows Mr Jenkins best. When the GP returns, she feels that a specialist opinion is required because she does not feel competent to make the relevant assessment of capacity and best interests. She contacts the local old age psychiatry department who send out a community psychiatric nurse (CPN) to assess the patient, having first suggested that the assessment of his capacity should be within the remit of the GP. The CPN agrees that Mr Jenkins is depressed, but says that his consultant colleague would have to assess capacity. After a further delay the consultant psychiatrist visits and agrees both that Mr Jenkins is depressed and that he lacks capacity to make decisions about treatment; she says that, in her opinion, covert medication would be in the best interests of Mr Jenkins, but suggests that the GP should make this decision because she knows Mr Jenkins best. The home wants a form to be signed to confirm a doctor's opinion; there is a further delay whilst the doctors negotiate who should sign the form. Mr Jenkins then receives covert medication and after two weeks his mood starts to improve. His appetite picks up and he becomes much brighter.

This case leads to a question about who should make any particular decision. The Code of Practice for the MCA is quite clear that: 'The person who assesses an individual's capacity to make a decision will usually be the person who is directly concerned with the individual at the time the decision needs to be made' (Department for Constitutional Affairs 2007, MCA Code of Practice, paragraph 4.38), and later it says that, 'The final decision about a person's capacity must be made by the person intending to make the decision or carry out the action of the person who lacks capacity' (Code of Practice, paragraph 4.42). There would be grounds for arguing that anyone from the family to the consultant could be regarded as the decision-maker and, therefore, as the person who should carry out the assessment of capacity. The decision to put Mr Jenkins on an antidepressant is obviously a medical one. But the decision to give the medication covertly is not so obviously medical. There may be pharmacological issues about how the tablet or capsule is crushed or diluted and so forth, but having established the route of administration, there is still the decision to give it covertly. Actually it could be argued that this decision is an ethical one. Perhaps the expertise required is that of an ethicist! Indeed, it seems to me very reasonable to argue that all clinical decisions are, at one and the same time, ethical. But if the central decision to be made is an ethical one – is it right or wrong to give Mr Jenkins covert medication? – then what are the grounds for arguing that the consultant psychiatrist is better placed than the nurse to make this decision? And could it not be said that the daughter is a better arbiter of what might be right or wrong for her father?

Once again, although the MCA defines good practice, there is a concern that it could lead to bureaucratic strife. In a sense the strife is no bad thing if it leads to clarity and is for the good of patients. However, it has also encouraged a tendency to uncertainty, which leads to the requirement that a further opinion should be sought. This makes for a more prolonged process of assessment when, in the past, decisions might have been swifter. A quick decision might be bad, but not inevitably so. It is not automatically clear that all this has been good for Mr Jenkins. First, he has had to undergo several assessments, where the reality is that the nurse and the family could have made the decision together. Second, it is not good that there has been a degree of therapeutic paralysis whilst bureaucratic processes have been worked out. The defence of the MCA is to say that these are mere problems of implementation of the Act. None the less, the MCA is inevitably a bureaucratic process and thereby encourages a sense of uncertainty, which it is worth considering.

The uncertainty can be considered in the light of the tension I am highlighting between the need to interfere with professional practice and the need to let judgements in health and social care be made in an unimpeded manner. Uncertainty may, as I suggested above, amount to 'therapeutic paralysis': clinicians may simply feel uncertain about whether they can proceed, or whether there is some other assessment that is required. This type of uncertainty is not merely about process. Rather, it reflects the feeling that capacity assessments, now enshrined in statute law, are technical or specialized. To this extent the uncertainty is negative.

Positive uncertainty: Pausing and best interests

There is, however, a positive type of uncertainty. Sometimes, it is good to pause. It can be on the side of patients. Important decisions about their lives should not (unless they must) be made quickly. Part of the reason for having a pause is precisely to allow the person, if possible, to be involved in decision-making. Inasmuch as the MCA encourages the positive uncertainty of the pause, it represents warranted interference in clinical care. This is especially so in the face of other pressures on clinicians, for instance to clear busy medical beds. The pause of the MCA is a necessary corrective to other bureaucratic pressures that militate against best quality patient care. Alternatively, the negative uncertainty, to do with following legal procedures relevant to assessment, is not unconditionally helpful.

Box 7.3 Mrs Krasinska

Mrs Krasinska, an 81-year-old widow, was admitted to a stroke unit some weeks ago. Her physical state is now stable, but she has a poor swallow. She had a pneumonia in the second week of her admission and she then developed a second chest infection which was quite severe. She survived, but it is clear that she is aspirating: food and drink are going into her lungs. A decision has to be made concerning artificial feeding, using a PEG tube. The treating medical team find it very difficult to assess her capacity to make this decision. The gastroenterologist who is called to discuss the PEG tube says he cannot understand what she says because of her dysarthric (slurred) speech and strong Polish accent. The speech and language therapist has been involved over the swallowing but she is also unable to help with communication. It is decided to involve an old age psychiatrist, since there is evidence of cognitive impairment.

At interview, Mrs Krasinska appears to understand the risks of aspirating, says she does not wish to die, but also says she would like to be able to continue to drink. She refuses to have a PEG tube. When water is put within her reach she goes to drink it, despite having just said she knows it might be dangerous. It is difficult to tell whether she is simply being unwise, which she is allowed to be under the MCA, or whether her contradictory statements and actions represent a deficit in terms of decision-making. The team feel they need more time to assess her. She continues to be given fluid by subcutaneous drip (i.e. through a small needle inserted under the skin). Two days later, Mrs Krasinska's nephew visits and she agrees to have a PEG tube inserted in the hope that she will gradually be able to drink by mouth again in the future if her condition improves. It is still not clear whether or not she has capacity, but the decision seems, in any event, to be in her best interests.

The case raises a number of points. As in the case of Mr Jenkins, the MCA leads, in a sense, to delays in the treatment of Mrs Krasinska.

But in this case, the delays seem helpful in that they have allowed a little more surety to develop concerning what might be best. At the start of the process, it would have seemed wrong to take Mrs Krasinska off against her wishes to have a PEG tube. By the end of the process she had come round to this way of thinking. The medical team had gone to some lengths to try to understand her and her wishes, as well as to evaluate her capacity and decision-making abilities in general. The whole process of seeking further opinions has meant that the decision about Mrs Krasinska's long-term care was made with greater consideration and in a way that allowed her to feel more in control.

In terms of ethical principles, we can see that the team have tried to respect the autonomy of Mrs Krasinska. They have also tried to act in a beneficent manner. In addition, they have been keen that, whatever decision was made, it should do no harm (that is, the principle of non-maleficence). The MCA prevented a rather paternalistic decision being made even if it also caused some delays.

Underlying tensions

The MCA allows people to appoint attorneys to act for them. There are two sorts of Lasting Powers of Attorney. One covers property and finance and the other covers welfare, which means both health and social decisions. It remains true, almost seven years after the Act came into effect, that relatively few welfare LPAs have been created. Fewer still have been put into effect. This may be a bureaucratic issue because people have complained about the complexity and cost associated with setting up a LPA. It could be, however, that, beyond the practicalities, there are deeper social and ethical issues. For instance, it may be that the demand for LPAs comes from a relatively narrow band of society, those who see autonomy as a crucial principle of liberal democracy and LPAs as a weapon to combat unfettered interference with what a person's true wishes might be. This view faces difficulties if, in fact, the population at large are more willing to accept the judgements of healthcare professionals. It might be that part of their willingness to accept a degree of future dependency stems from a tacit presumption that the decisions that will have to be made might be too taxing for them even to consider asking someone near to them to have to make. Or, it may more simply be that people feel more uncertainty around what may or may not happen in the future. There seem to be a number of barriers to successful advance care planning (Robinson *et al.* 2013).

In other words, it might be that the public accepts the underlying need for a degree of professional autonomy without interference. Optimistically, there may be a belief that professionals will make good decisions. But we know that this is not always the case. One question is whether the MCA helps professionals to make decisions, or whether it might make them more tentative in their decision-making, which in turn might lead to a loss of confidence in their abilities to make good decisions. Of course, it can be argued that the current state of affairs involves too much power in the hands of professionals, so that anything that might encourage more shared decision-making would be a good thing.

The MCA also allows Advance Decisions to Refuse Treatment (ADRTs). But ADRTs are not legally binding if they are not valid and if they are not applicable. To be valid they must be made in an appropriate manner. For instance, if the matter is to do with life-sustaining treatment, then the advance refusal must be in writing, must be signed and witnessed. Applicability, however, is a nebulous notion. It suggests that if anything has happened which could be taken to imply that the person might have or would have changed their minds, then the advance refusal is no longer applicable. So, for instance, if a person has stipulated that they wish to have no medical interference, but they have then visited their doctor on numerous occasions seeking medical help, it could be argued that the advance refusal of treatment is not applicable. Similarly, if an ADRT was made by someone unaware that, some years later, an effective treatment was going to emerge, then the advance refusal could be deemed inapplicable. The tension is again between the unfettered exercise of clinical judgement and the legal process being used to control medical decisions. The reality is that a line has to be drawn. There will be areas in which it is right and proper that the professionals should be able to make reasonable judgements without going through bureaucratic processes. But there will be other areas where the bureaucratic process is not only helpful but a manifestation of a respect for human rights. The provision for advance refusals of treatment is clearly meant to swing the pendulum in favour of patients having more say in terms of what happens to them. A good effect of the MCA is that advance care planning, when it is done at its best, involves careful discussion and negotiation between the parties concerned. The trouble is that, as yet, this still does not occur commonly. It may be, however, given the complexity of the task, that there simply are not the resources to allow this type of careful planning for everyone.

One of the innovations of the MCA has been to give more of a voice to those who are 'unbefriended' through the use of Independent Mental Capacity Advocates (IMCAs). That is, where the person who lacks capacity has no family or friends or other non-professional carers to support them and where a significant decision about healthcare or where the person resides is being made, the Act says that an IMCA must be appointed. The ability of the IMCA to spend some time looking in detail at what might be in the person's best interests is often very helpful. Those who have used IMCAs to help make best interests decisions have tended to be favourably impressed. There is a worry, however, that the use of IMCAs is patchy and, in particular, that the use of IMCAs for serious medical treatments is relatively much lower than their use for questions about place of residence. This obviously needs some research, but it would not be at all implausible to suggest that the problem stems precisely from the tension that I have been highlighting. Perhaps it is still the case that IMCAs are seen as an unwarranted interference in matters that are clearly medical and should remain solely medical. Alternatively, most simply, the MCA has simply not been understood properly and this represents a failure in terms of implementation. Or, in a more complicated fashion, it may be that the lack of use of IMCAs for serious medical treatments is again a reflection of the tension, on the one hand, between the natural wish of doctors to get on with treating their patients in the patient's best interests as a manifestation of the therapeutic relationship (that is, a personal thing) and, on the other, interference by the *polis* (a public matter).

Deprivations and restrictions

This tension is perhaps seen more obviously in the response of practitioners to the *Deprivation of Liberty Safeguards*. I shall not go over the bureaucratic details of the Deprivation of Liberty Safeguards (DoLS), which have been set out very thoroughly elsewhere (Welsh and Keeling 2013). The need for DoLS came about following the well-known Bournewood judgement, which involved a man with autism (HL) who was held in Bournewood Hospital informally, that is without the provisions of the Mental Health Act 1983 (MHA), but without any intention that he should be able to leave. His foster parents were not even allowed to visit. Having passed through different courts in England, with conflicting judgements, the case finally went to the European Court and the Deprivation of Liberty Safeguards resulted from the judgement in October 2004 in connection with the European Convention on Human Rights. The decision regarding the young man with autism (HL) was that people can only be deprived of their liberty if there is a process set out in law with safeguards to prevent arbitrary detention. And the European Court said that there should be speedy access to a court to review the detention if this were to occur. In short, you are not allowed to deprive someone of their liberty unless there are legal safeguards in place.

This raises the question, what is a deprivation of liberty? The courts have said that only they can decide this, but that it will depend on the particular circumstances of the case and there can be no definitive definition of deprivation of liberty. It is necessary to consider all the factors that might contribute to a deprivation of liberty and it cannot be said that there is any one factor that would decide matters.

The confusion is that the MCA allows the use of restraint (in Sections 5 and 6). Restraint can only be used if there is a reasonable belief that the person lacks capacity and that the act of restraint will be in the person's best interests. But any such restraint must be proportionate to the harm that is being avoided by using the restraint. In connection with deprivation of liberty, therefore, the European Court said that the distinction between a deprivation of and restriction upon liberty 'is merely one of degree or intensity and not one of nature or substance' (Ministry of Justice 2008, DoLS Code of Practice 2.2). It has been suggested that it is helpful to see restriction of liberty as being on a scale, which eventually moves into deprivation of liberty depending on the concrete circumstances of the individual case.

In the case of *JE and DE v Surrey County Council*, which was a high court judgement on 29 December 2006, the judge, Mr Justice Munby, accepted that DE, who was a man in a care home, was free to leave, free to use the communal garden, could telephone, was taken out by staff and had never tried to leave, nor expressed a wish to leave, although he had said that he wished to live with his wife, JE, but had never requested to go immediately with JE when she left. The judge also accepted that the staff in the home listened to, supported and reassured Mr DE. Nevertheless, Mr DE was recorded as having said 'you are holding me against my civil rights, all I want to do is to be with my wife'. The judge said that the crucial issue was:

> whether DE was or was not, is or is not, 'free to leave'. And I agree... DE was not and is not 'free to leave', and was and is, in that sense, completely under the control of [Surrey County Council], because...it was and is [Surrey County Council] who decide the essential matters where DE can live, whether he can leave and whether he can be with JE. (paragraph 117)

In other words, Mr Justice Munby accepted that DE had 'a very substantial degree of freedom...a very substantial degree of contact with the outside world', and was not subjected to any invasive degree of control as in the case of HL. For instance, there was no physical or chemical restraint (paragraph 114). Nevertheless, the judge felt that DE was deprived of his liberty because he was not 'free to leave'.

The judgement of Mr Justice Munby is helpfully clear. The notion of being 'free to leave', however, does not really take the debate about whether something is merely a restriction or an actual deprivation of liberty much further. The difference between someone who has been abducted and secretly imprisoned, or someone who languishes in a concentration camp, on the one hand, and, on the other, the confused elderly patient who has just undergone hip surgery, or even the elderly care home resident who thinks that her parents will be shortly expecting her home and that she must, therefore, leave, could not be greater. None is 'free to leave'. They would all, therefore, seemingly be deprived of their liberty, but this seems nonsensical.

In the original judgement of HL the European Court objected to the exercise of 'complete and effective control over his care and his movements' (paragraph 91 of *HL v United Kingdom* (2004) 40 EHRR 761). We gain a little more insight into what 'complete and effective control' might mean when the European judges expanded this to say that the professionals had 'the clear intention…to exercise strict control over his assessment, treatment, contacts and notably movement and residence; the applicant would only be released… as and when those professionals considered it appropriate'. So complete control means control over such matters as with whom the person comes into contact and it implies that no one else will have any say-so in when or whether the person is released from the detention. We can see that these issues would apply to the abduction and the concentration camp, but would not necessarily apply to the orthopaedic ward or the care home.

A further important case has been that of P (also known as MIG) and Q (also known as MEG). This went to the Court of Appeal in 2011 (CoA [2011] EWCA Civ 190). MIG and MEG were two girls aged 17 and 18 who were cared for by the local authority. They both had learning disabilities. MIG lived in a family home, whereas MEG lived in a group home with four residents. MIG was subjected to continuous supervision and control in order to meet her care needs, but she was not on any medication and there were no particular social restrictions and she was able to attend college.

MEG, on the other hand, lived in a small group home having been found incapable of independent living. Her mother was unable to care for her and MEG was not allowed to go out alone, but had no restrictions on her contacts and she was able both to attend college and to live a lively social life. In both cases the court found that they were not deprived of their liberty. The court said that a deprivation of liberty had three elements: an objective element, a subjective element and that the confinement was 'imputable' to the state. In other words, these laws are only concerned with cases where the state in effect brings about the putative deprivation of liberty. In considering the objective element, the court said that this did not depend on whether or not the person was happy, because that only relates to whether or not the arrangements will be in the person's best interests. Nevertheless, the court said that whether the person was objecting to their confinement and the degree of conflict that this entailed would be very relevant to the objective element. In addition, if medication, in particular antipsychotic drugs or other tranquillizers, were being used this would tend to push the judgement towards the finding of a deprivation of liberty. The question is whether the drugs would be used to suppress the person's liberty to express his or her wishes. The judges also considered that the normality of the arrangements should be taken into account too. That is, it is harder to conceive that someone living in a normal house is deprived of liberty compared to a person in a large institution.

The factors outlined in the MIG and MEG case, as well as in the earlier cases, do help to sketch where a deprivation of liberty may start and where a mere restriction of liberty ends. Nonetheless, the underlying tension concerning ordinary care and interference by the state is still present.

In his seminal work, George Agich (2003) talked about the difference between dependence and autonomy in old age, thinking specifically of people who live in long-term care. He made the point that dependence and autonomy are opposite sides of the same coin. Our autonomy is partly exercised through our dependence. In other words, my ability to go on holiday and travel where I like is only possible through my dependence on more people than I can probably count, from travel agents to hotel staff to air traffic control. I achieve my autonomy through my dependence. The balance between autonomy and dependence changes through life. Agich says this:

> Autonomy fundamentally importantly involves the way individuals live their daily lives; it is found in the nooks and crannies of everyday experience; it is found in the way that individuals interact and not exclusively in the idealised paradigm of choice or decision-making that dominates ethical analysis. (2003, p.165)

He goes on to say that for older people, as for us all, autonomy is properly understood in the context of 'essential inter-relationship with others and the world' (p.174). As I get older, that is, there is a gradual increase in terms of my dependence on other people. If I have particular diseases, from physical diseases to organic mental diseases such as dementia, my dependence increases in particular ways. My liberty to pursue my autonomous wishes inevitably decreases. In other words, part of normal life and normal ageing is that there is a restriction of my liberty in one way or another. Now, it seems to me that a deprivation of liberty is something really quite extreme and should not in any way be confused with care that is normal and necessary in conditions themselves unexceptional in the context of ageing.

Conclusion

In a rather beautiful passage in *The Needs of Strangers*, Michael Ignatieff wrote the following:

> Rights language offers a rich vernacular for the claims an individual may make on or against the collectivity, but it is relatively impoverished as a means of expressing individuals' needs *for* the collectivity. It can only express our human ideal of fraternity as a mutual respect for rights, and it can only defend the claim to be treated with dignity in terms of our common identity as rights-bearing creatures. Yet we are more than rights-bearing creatures,

and there is more to respect in a person than his rights. (Ignatieff 1984, p.13)

We could put this by saying we have a need *for the polis* even if, at the same time, we have rights to protect us against the demands *of the polis*. Ignatieff went on to say:

It is because fraternity, love, longing, dignity, respect, cannot be specified as rights that we ought to specify them as needs and seek, with the blunt institutional procedures at our disposal, to make their satisfaction a routine practice. (pp.13–14)

In other words, there are some things which are not rights but which nevertheless we should be seeking through our communities. My conclusion is not that the MCA is bureaucratic and it is not that DoLS are unnecessary. In fact, I think that the MCA is helpful. But it is enacted against a background in which there must already be in place certain values and virtues, which are necessary if the care of vulnerable people is to be as good as possible. Nonetheless, when bureaucracy bears down too heavily on professional practice, it puts at risk the primacy of the interpersonal relationship and the chances that from this will emerge compassion, concern and creativity. It is a necessary feature of liberal democracy that the law should protect those who are vulnerable. But something can be lost, and the type of fiduciary relationship, based on trust, which constitutes good clinical practice, is itself vulnerable. It is also valued and not only by health professionals.

When all is said and done, however, the aim of the *polis*, according to Plato, is the common good. The state has a vital role to play in terms of directing the people through its laws. And one purpose of the *polis* is to direct its citizens towards the good. To this end, the words of Martin Luther King, Jr on receiving his Honorary Doctorate of Civil Law from Newcastle University on 13 November 1967 seem apposite:

And so while the law may not change the hearts of men, it does change the habits of men if vigorously enforced, and through changes in habits, pretty soon attitudinal changes will take place and even the heart may be changed in the process. (King 1967)[9]

---

9   Since writing this chapter, there have been two important developments. First, the House of Lords Select Committee on the Mental Capacity Act 2005 published its *Mental Capacity Act 2005: Post-legislative Scrutiny* (House of Lords 2014). It found that there had been a failure to embed the MCA in everyday practice. Arguably, the concerns expressed in this chapter would feed into that failure, but would also call into question the likely success of their Lordships' answer, which is to increase the bureaucracy by creating an independent body to oversee the implementation of the Act. They also found that the Deprivation of Liberty Safeguards were not working and they suggested they should be replaced.

    Secondly, there has recently been a Supreme Court judgement on the cases of MIG and MEG, with their Lordships, by a majority, reaching the conclusion that they were deprived of liberty. The judgement suggests a single test for deprivation of liberty, namely whether the person is under continuous supervision and control and is not free to leave. See: *P (by his litigation friend the Official Solicitor) (Appellant) v Cheshire West and Chester Council and another (Respondents); P and Q (by their litigation friend, the Official Solicitor) (Appellants) v Surrey County Council (Respondent)* [2014] UKSC 19 On appeal from [2011] EWCA Civ 1257; [2011] EWCA Civ 190.

CHAPTER 8

Incapacity and Mental Disorder

Introduction

In the spirit of questioning, my intention in this chapter is to raise questions about the link between mental disorder and mental incapacity. I wish both to raise some questions and to point in the direction of answers located in the real world. But this is not to say that the answers will make life cosy. In fact, the answers might make things more complicated. Nevertheless, I think that understanding the complexity a little better might, perhaps, make us feel more at home in the world.

So, I intend to do the following: first, I shall present a rationale for the distinction between the Mental Capacity Act (MCA) and the Mental Health Act (MHA); second, to make things real, I shall consider an albeit fictional medical case and a real legal one; third, I shall try to face the philosophical confusion that emerges; fourth, I shall try to introduce some philosophical clarity, even if this means seeing things in a complicated way; finally, I shall summarize by using a slogan derived from the philosopher Mary Midgley, namely 'One world, but a big one' (Midgley 2001).

The legal rationale

In a seminar organized by the Making Decisions Alliance, before the MCA came into being in 2005, Lord Filkin summarized the difference between the MCA and the MHA. He said that different principles applied to the two bills. The MCA is to do with making decisions. The MHA is to do with risk. This was stated fairly clearly and I think it is what we all know intuitively. Lord Filkin went on to say that the basis of the MCA is, obviously, the issue of incapacity and what must be done in the face of incapacity. The guiding principle is to act in the best interests of the patient. This remains true whoever is making the decision, whether it be the Court of Protection, someone holding a Lasting Power of Attorney, or the family carer. On the other hand, the MHA is concerned with matters to do with safety and the provisions for compulsory treatment and detention. It was also made clear that once we enter the territory of issues around safety, detention and compulsory treatment, then the MHA should 'trump' the MCA.

I want to go back now to a debate in the pages of the *Psychiatric Bulletin* in 1998, when George Szmukler and Frank Holloway wrote:

> The message is as follows, though ill, those with a mental disorder are somehow different. That is why they require separate legislation. They may be treated against their will irrespective of whether they have the capacity to consent to treatment. This suggests a pervasive and disturbing notion that 'mental' patients somehow are incapable of possessing a full degree of autonomy; mental disorder automatically diminishes the sufferer; he or she is not a complete 'person'. (Szmukler and Holloway 1998)

In a response to the Szmukler–Holloway article, Fulford and Sayce (1998) accepted that there was something discriminatory in the difference between the way physical and mental illness is regarded under the law, but were concerned, if I might paraphrase, that a simple solution, doing away with mental health legislation altogether, even if it got rid of one complexity, would lead to another complexity, namely the complexity of determining capacity in the face of mental illness. Again to paraphrase, they argued that whilst the notion of 'capacity' looks as if it might be straightforward, in fact, in the context of mental illness, it is very difficult, and that is because the whole notion of mental disorder (or mental illness) is much more complicated and, therefore, difficult to deal with, than the notion of bodily or physical disorder. They said:

> If we assume that judgements of incapacity can be made with no less difficulty for mental disorders than for bodily disorders, then we will be at risk of either including those who should be excluded or excluding those who should be included. (Fulford and Sayce 1998, p.667)

Thus, whilst the MHA has a broad definition of mental disorder and whilst, therefore, it looks like it might be over-inclusive in terms of allowing that people with capacity can be treated against their wishes, Fulford suggests that there is a danger in going the other way. That is, there is a danger of over-exclusive legislation, which tries to keep out those people with mental illnesses who have capacity. But, Fulford is suggesting, some of these people might benefit from treatment, even against their wishes. Now, this last statement is arguable, but I am not going to argue for it, although I think I shall be making comments pertinent to the debate.

Luckily, since 1998 there has been some empirical work to inform this debate. I am aware of two papers in the *Journal of Mental Health Law*, by Bellhouse and colleagues, which have considered capacity-based mental health legislation and its impact on clinical practice (Bellhouse *et al*. 2003a, 2003b). The sample they studied comprised 49 individuals. In the first paper, which concerned admission to hospital, a significant relationship was found between having a psychotic illness and incapacity (Bellhouse *et al*. 2003a). Fourteen of sixteen people unable to consent had a psychotic disorder. The overall conclusions from both papers included the following points. Although there was a considerable overlap, capacity-based mental health legislation would not result in exactly the same people being liable to be detained as under the current MHA. Two of ten detained people in the study were capable of consenting to admission. One of these might have been detainable if risk to others were considered sufficient grounds for overriding a competent adult. This raises the question whether it would be better to use criminal law rather than mental health law to detain someone who poses a risk to others, but who is capable with respect to the decision about admission.

The first of these papers concluded with the suggestion that the data supported the use of capacity assessments as part of the criteria for compulsion: 'As well as a strong ethical argument in support of such change, there is also no reason to think that such change might be unworkable or have disastrous consequences' (Bellhouse *et al.* 2003a, p.22).

It would be possible to spend some time simply discussing the details and arguments raised by these two important papers and I apologize for giving them short shrift, but I note a slight contradiction, perhaps, when I read the concluding paragraphs of the second paper where it says: 'It may be, though, that the correlation between incapacity and psychotic symptoms would leave people suffering from non-psychotic disorders at risk of suicide and other adverse health outcomes' (Bellhouse *et al.* 2003b, p.36).

The first conclusion favours the Szmukler-Holloway view (we should use incapacity as the criterion for compulsory treatment); the second favours the Fulford-Sayce view (we should stick with the devil we know, namely mental disorder). So, maybe empirical research does not always give definitive answers to value-laden questions. Well, let us retreat to a clinical case.

Two cases

Mrs Sengupta has dementia. It is moderately severe. She has been wandering in the street once or twice and there are other concerns at home. The old age psychiatrist invites Mrs Sengupta to the hospital and she comes fairly willingly. After a few hours, however, she starts to become agitated. She wants to go home. But she is disorientated in both time and place. There is prior evidence of poor self-care. Mrs Sengupta starts banging on the doors and hitting the staff nurse. The staff nurse finds the doctor and says that the MHA will have to be used in order both to detain and treat Mrs Sengupta. The doctor is disinclined to use the MHA and says that the team should continue to use the provision of the MCA because the issue is Mrs Sengupta's lack of capacity.

At some point, it might be agreed, the MHA should be used, but what level of aggression on the part of Mrs Sengupta, or physical restraint on the part of the staff, warrants passing from the MCA to the MHA?

These are important problems and the story shows some of the conceptual difficulties. It also demonstrates the working of the legal rationale that we discussed before. When the issue is merely capacity and trying to do what is best for Mrs Sengupta, it is reasonable to use capacity legislation. Once we move, to use the language of Lord Filkin, into the territory of *safety, overt detention and compulsory treatment*, the MHA trumps mental capacity or incapacity legislation.

Let me leave this point by simply highlighting the way in which, whilst the law makes a distinction between incapacity and mental illness and whilst that distinction has some intuitive face value, at the coalface it is a matter of fairly fine judgements. These are not just judgements about matters of fact – they are judgements of value, with all sorts of things coming into play, such as the quality of Mrs Sengupta's distress, the attitudes of her family, the circumstances of the ward, to name but a few.

I want now to turn to a legal case in order to encourage my philosophical thoughts. It is the case of *B v Croydon Health Authority*, heard in the Court of Appeal in 1994 (*B v Croydon Health Authority* [1995] Fam 133). B was a 24-year-old woman with a diagnosis of borderline personality disorder, coupled with post-traumatic stress disorder. Her symptoms included depression and a compulsion to self-harm. She was detained under Section 3 of the MHA. Once detained, she had no means of hurting herself, so she virtually stopped eating and the question that arose was whether she could be force-fed.

To summarize, there were two potential questions for the judges. First, there was a question about whether she might lack capacity and then, secondly, there was a question about whether force-feeding her would count as treatment for her mental disorder. The issue of lack of capacity was not formally decided, although the judges indicated they thought she probably did not have it.

Lord Justice Hoffmann instead made a decision about the issue of treatment for mental disorder. The key section in the MHA (1983) is section 63, which (having excluded treatment falling within sections 57 and 58) states the following:

> The consent of a patient shall not be required for any medical treatment given to him for the mental disorder from which he is suffering…if the treatment is given by or under the direction of the responsible medical officer.

Council representing B suggested the very reasonable argument that, since everyone agreed that the only effective treatment for her diagnosis was psychoanalytic psychotherapy, force-feeding was not a treatment for her mental disorder. He said that giving the food might be a prerequisite to a treatment for her mental disorder or it might be treatment for a consequence of her mental disorder, but it was not treatment of the disorder itself. Concerning this, Lord Justice Hoffmann said:

> This is a powerful submission. But I have come to the conclusion that it is too atomistic. It requires every individual element of the treatment being given to the patient to be directed to his mental condition. But in my view this test applies only to the treatment as a whole.

Hoffmann then referred to the definition of 'medical treatment' contained in section 145(1) of the MHA, which includes 'nursing…care, habilitation and rehabilitation under medical supervision'. Lord Justice Hoffmann accepted that there must be a treatment for her 'psychopathic disorder' otherwise it would not be lawful to detain her. But he said that it did not follow that every act which forms a part of that treatment within the wide definition of section 145(1) 'must in itself be likely to alleviate or prevent a deterioration of that disorder'. The remarkable thing, I think, in the statements by Lord Justice Hoffmann is the way in which he regards the 'powerful submission' of B's counsel as being *'too atomistic'*. I also like the way he spoke of *'treatment as a whole'*.

Philosophical confusion

I wish now to consider how all of these issues can become confused. But my argument is essentially very simple, because it states that the issues we are dealing with appear confused at times because they are complex. Philosophical clarity comes from seeing the complexity.

One way to make ourselves confused would be to consider the various ways in which mental disorder and mental incapacity might be related. 'Mental disorder' is now defined in the 1983 Act as 'any disorder or disability of the mind'. Hence, mental incapacity is simply a subtype of 'mental disorder'.

But if this were the case, why should we not always have used the MHA to deal with mental incapacity when there were significant dangers that warranted detention or treatment? One answer is that some incapacitated patients are compliant and, therefore, it does not appear that the MHA needs to be used. The result is that they lack the safeguards of those detained under the MHA, who are mainly psychotic. This is the 'Bournewood gap' identified by Lord Steyn in the famous Bournewood case (which we met in Chapter 7), where he said: 'There can be no justification for not giving to compliant incapacitated patients the same quality and degree of protection as is given to patients admitted under the Act of 1983' (*R v Bournewood Community and Mental Health NHS Trust*, ex parte L [1998] 3 AllER 289). But I wonder whether Lord Steyn was misinformed, even though his conclusion seems, at first blush, so reasonable. Early in his judgement he said: 'Diagnostically there is usually no or virtually no difference between…[compliant incapacitated patients] and patients compulsorily admitted under the Act of 1983.'

This is, to me at least, not obviously true. To put it crudely, young psychotic patients look very different compared with old people with dementia. If you think they all have the same diagnosis, you are likely to think they should all be treated in the same way. But this is where confusion starts to emerge, because of the complexity.

On the one hand, we can think of mental incapacity as being a subset of mental disorder. On the other hand, at least in the field of dementia, we might wish to think of incapacity in much more organic terms. Dementia, after all, is an organic disorder and it is tempting to regard incapacity resulting from an 'organic' disorder as being markedly different from the un-understandable psychotic experiences of those people with 'functional' illnesses. Hence the possibility that we can assess mental incapacity in an objective way using objective tests, whether these be clinical tests or legal tests; whereas functional illnesses are more complicated precisely because the diagnoses are more value-laden. In short, cognitive tests of capacity make capacity look like a more straightforward (objective) concept.

So, with all due respect to Lord Steyn, from the diagnostic point of view, one might wish to represent incapacity and mental disorder as two quite separate things. This would give some rationale to the need for two separate acts of parliament, even if the Mental 'Disorder' Act eventually trumps the Mental 'Capacity' Act.

When I read the Bournewood judgement in full I was struck by the careful consideration given to section 131(1) of the Act of 1983 and to the background to that section. It states:

> Nothing in this Act shall be construed as preventing a patient who requires treatment for mental disorder from being admitted to any hospital or mental nursing home in pursuance of arrangements made in that behalf and without any application, order or direction rendering him liable to be detained under this Act... (MHA 1983, Section 131(1))

Lord Gough traced this section back through the 1959 Act to the recommendations of the Percy Commission of 1957. The Percy Commission (1957) had recommended that compulsory detention should only be employed where it was necessary. In paragraph 289 they made it clear that they wished to see 'the need for care' and 'the justification for compulsion' as two quite separate questions. In paragraph 291 they suggested that the assumption that compulsory powers must be used unless the patient can express a positive desire for treatment should be abandoned and replaced by 'the offer of care without deprivation of liberty, to all who need it and are not unwilling to receive it'. This seems very humane and it got rid of the previous situation in which incapacitated compliant patients had to be detained, because they could not agree to treatment.

The thought I am pursuing here is that there is something laudable in the distinction between 'the need for care' and 'the justification for compulsion'. This might, arguably, be another reason for keeping the notions of incapacity and mental disorder separate. By and large, people with incapacity need only ordinary care. Well, it might also be argued that the same is true much of the time for people with mental disorder. But they sometimes need extraordinary care when the issues of safety, detention and compulsory treatment raise their ugly heads. Similarly, these ugly heads sometimes appear for people with incapacity. But maybe it is only at this point that they should be regarded as having a mental disorder. In which case, not all incapacity is mental illness.

I should quickly add here that I am not proposing these ideas as arguments I wish to defend to the hilt. My intention is rather to raise the conceptual complexities. One of the conceptual complexities is the whole issue of normal ageing. When I am 90 years old, how much incapacity should be regarded as normal? Similarly, there are well known conceptual difficulties around the notion of 'illness' (Fulford 1989). Thus, it could be said, as regards illness, the broad definition of 'mental disorder' in the 1983 MHA simply went too far, as shown by a grandmother's reluctance to be regarded as ill just because she no longer remembers the exact date.

Here is another outlandish suggestion: perhaps mental disorder is a subset of mental incapacity. After all, to have a mental disorder is something rather special. To be incapacitated to some degree, it seems to me, is ubiquitous. For instance, I have never fully understood my mortgage arrangements. Making difficult decisions is commonplace. Someone might object to the idea that all mental disorder involves incapacity on the grounds that people with mental illness pass tests of capacity. But so what? Perhaps the tests are not subtle enough. Perhaps, for the most part, lacking full capacity does not matter. It does not matter that I do not fully understand my mortgage, but my understanding is not helped by even a mild degree of dysphoria. Pertinent here are questions about 'disorder' and normal sadness or normal elation.

These are not the only ways in which mental disorder and mental incapacity might relate, but it would take too long to examine every possibility and I am more interested in highlighting the potential for confusion in this whole area. If there is confusion, it is because of conceptual complexity.

Philosophical clarity

As already suggested, philosophical clarity comes from seeing the complexity. At the start of this chapter I suggested that the point of raising questions was to direct us towards a better understanding of the world. And I think that the philosophical, that is conceptual, arguments we have been toying with already point us towards a clearer vision, once we can see it, inasmuch as they show us where the conceptual complexities arise.

They arise around the concepts of mental disorder, mental illness, mental incapacity, normal ageing, ordinary care and the like. One of the subliminal themes is the importance of values. We have already toyed with these ideas in Chapter 6. In his earlier work, Fulford (1989) helped to establish the thought that values are pervasive in clinical practice. Diagnosis is rife with evaluative decisions: where does normal sadness turn into depression? This theme has been built upon by Sadler (2004) in his examination of the evaluative nature of the American *Diagnostic and Statistical Manual* (DSM). This was before the furore over the new edition (DSM-5), which seems to have created a number of new conditions that some would argue reflect normal behaviours. Fulford's thought has developed into values-based practice, which attempts both to make values explicit – to get them onto the table alongside the facts of evidence-based practice – and to provide a framework within which to consider values and to negotiate, through good communication, when values are diverse and disputed (Fulford 2004).

It would not take much to persuade you that values are important in connection with mental disorder and mental illness; but part of the simplifying trickery surrounding mental incapacity is the suggestion that this is *more* factual, reflecting the organic nature of mental incapacity. This trickery is inherent in the legal and clinical tests for various types of incapacity. It may well be that the trickery is necessary and it may well serve a useful function, but it should not persuade us into thinking that the concepts are simple.

In fact, these concepts do not have clear boundaries, but nor are clear boundaries needed in order for them to be usable. To be usable they must fit into *patterns of practice*. That is, the justification for using the notion of mental disorder or mental incapacity will come from the various ways in which these notions fit into our overall patterns of practice. Rather than pursue this in any detail, let me just derive one thing from it. It seems to suggest that what we need is the whole picture, rather than simply parts of it. Hence, if you ask me which of the pictures I have sketched correctly depicts the relationship between mental disorder, or mental illness and incapacity, my answer is none of them.

You may remember that I said I would leave the thoughts from Lord Hoffmann's judgement in the B case hanging in the air. He was talking about the treatment of mental disorder and he criticized B's counsel for taking a view that was 'too atomistic'. He said we must consider 'treatment as a whole'. This seems to me entirely right. We need to see the whole picture and it is a picture of the world. It is here that I should like to use as a slogan the title of a chapter by Mary Midgley: 'One world, but a big one' (Midgley 2001, pp.122–9)!

Mental disorder, mental illness and mental incapacity intermingle and interconnect in this world picture. It is a picture into which Bill Fulford's emphasis on values in addition to facts must appear. It is a picture in which physical illness is not unrelated to mental incapacity and is not unrelated to mental illness. Furthermore, if it is a picture of the world, what should we leave out? Genetics is relevant to mental illness and mental incapacity. But the family is relevant, too, because of social relations and psychological dependencies. And this brings in the psychopathology of everyday life, so we are also talking about personality, as well as the psychopathology of mental illness. But these factors operate within a field of cultural traditions, laws, moral theories, religious beliefs and aesthetic appreciation. There is no limit, it is one world but a big one.

Conclusion

Well, but what is the link between incapacity and mental disorder? These concepts are linked by our appreciation of them within the context of this complex and big world. In other words, we are the link as people-in-the-world, whether we are patients, service users, psychiatrists, police officers or imams. What counts, therefore, will be the way we, as people-in-the-world, negotiate our way through this complexity. Inevitably we shall do this according to our patterns of practice, which we mentioned in the Introduction.

What guides these patterns of practice? The answer is, I think, almost everything. We are, of course, guided by the law. But we are also guided by professional judgements and professional ethics, which will determine, in particular cases, whether we are over-inclusive or over-exclusive in our application of criteria for assessing capacity. In addition, our personal *values, beliefs and intuitions* will make us tend to act this way rather than that. But these personal patterns will be set within the context of cultural values and social norms. This is certainly not nice and clear-cut and it leaves open the possibility of mistakes being made. But it seems to me it is the true picture. Our explanations of how things are, in psychiatry especially, cannot always afford to be simple. Judgements will have to be made against a background of complex interrelationships between facts, values, beliefs and intuitions.

I draw some comfort from, and will end with, a quotation from Mary Midgley in which she says:

> Of course simplicity is one aim of explanation. Of course we need parsimony. But it is no use being parsimonious unless you

are relevant. Explanations must be complex enough to do the particular work that they are there for, to answer the questions that are actually arising. There are always many alternative ways of simplifying things and we have to choose between them. The kind of parsimony that is too mean to deal with the points that really need explaining is not economy but futile miserliness. For any particular problem, we need a solution that sorts out the particular complications that puzzle us, not one that ignores them because they are untidy. (Midgley 2001, p.8)

I hope that being aware of the complexity is not a matter of ignoring the untidiness, but is a matter of being open to it. Being open to complexity, it seems to me, is likely to make clinical decisions better, if more difficult. We must hope for an optimal legal framework, but by its nature the framework is unlikely to capture the complexity and, in any case, it is only one facet of the patterns of practice that guide our clinical judgements. What is required, to understand the complex relationship between mental illness and mental incapacity and the like, is a perspicuous view of our patterns of practice. Our judgements must be based, as part of a complex practice, not on the application of a simple rule but on a reaction in particular circumstances. These circumstances may well involve disputed and diverse values, which will need to be negotiated. In Mrs Sengupta's case the doctor and the nurses will need to struggle through the thoughts about whether or not to use the MHA or whether the MCA is sufficient. The key is that this reaction to the particular circumstances – also our intuitions and background beliefs – must be shaped by the right sort of moral environment. To start with, this environment requires that we are open to discussing values and to accepting that sometimes others will hold different values. The environment must encourage the right sort of discussions. The struggle conceptually and legally is to create that environment. But it is made by multifarious factors, by everything that combines to shape our being-in-the-world and our being-with-others. The difficulty for the law is that it can influence the moral environment, but the moral environment, which in turn shapes the law, is based on a broader conception of the world.

PART IV

Palliative and Supportive Care

CHAPTER 9

Beyond Hypercognitivism

Introduction

It is too easy in the severer stages of dementia to regard the individual as lacking in personhood because of the marked deficits in recall memory. Taking an alternative view, that people with even severe dementia maintain emotional, relational and aesthetic aspects of personhood, encourages the thought that they are deserving of good quality palliative care. This chapter sets out philosophical support, from the broader view of personhood we have already discussed in Chapter 3, for good quality palliative care in dementia. It does this by considering the notion of 'human consciousness' (over against 'self-consciousness'). This builds on the earlier idea (again in Chapter 3) that our mindedness involves the external world. Good quality palliative care will take into account the broader understanding of what it is to be a person with dementia.

Hypercognitivism

When Stephen Post introduced, in 1995, the term 'hypercognitive' he had in view 'a persistent bias against the deeply forgetful that is especially pronounced in modern philosophical accounts of the 'person" (Post 2006, p.231). He stated: 'When the capacity to seek meaning in the midst of decline gives way to more advanced dementia…then the experience of the person must be understood in relational and affective terms rather than in narrowly cognitive ones' (Post 2000, p.85). Post has amply defended his position in his numerous writings over many years; he does not require my support. Nonetheless, in this chapter I wish to add a plank to the argument, which I hope might be seen as a tribute to Post's humane work.

In part, this work, of necessity, must be negative. For it involves combating the tendency amongst some philosophers to undermine the moral standing of people with dementia by denying them the ascription of personhood. There is, however, a positive message, which is that people with severe dementia deserve good quality palliative care. This can be regarded as having two aspects. First, palliative care involves accepting that some treatments are unnecessary because there is no hope of cure. The person should certainly not be burdened by aggressive or invasive treatments. Second, it should involve a change in approach and emphasis. In large measure, this will involve attention to the social and physical environment, as well as to issues of spirituality.

In an inspiring passage Post (2000, p.107) describes his vision thus:

> A new form of hospice for patients with advanced [dementia] would revolve around the concept of 'being with' rather than 'doing to' patients…, even if they have some years to live… Efforts to enhance emotional, relational, and esthetic well-being would, under such a plan, be enhanced in ways that involve family members, providing them with a sense of meaning and purpose. Through music, movement therapy, relaxation, and touch, such efforts support patients' remaining capacities. Connections with nature through a beautiful and open environment fit under this rubric, as can spiritual support.

In what follows I shall add philosophical support to the idea that beyond the hypercognitive there is plenty of room for an 'emotional, relational, and esthetic' understanding of personhood. But of course the reason for laying down this philosophical plank is to support the demand for better palliative care for people with severe dementia. And it is worth emphasizing Post's acknowledgement that severe dementia may last some years: we are not just talking about terminal care (Hughes 2005).

In focusing on a *philosophical* approach, I shall not consider the ever-increasing empirical evidence that supports the proposition that personhood persists in dementia. Much of the work of Tom Kitwood (1997) presupposed this proposition. Subsequently, the work of Steve Sabat (2001) has demonstrated how the self can be undermined or supported in people with dementia. In different ways, many workers in this field are able to give accounts to support the proposition of persisting personhood (Aquilina and Hughes 2006; Downs, Clare and Mackenzie 2006; Oppenheimer 2006; Sabat 2006; Snyder 2006).

Human consciousness

I shall start the philosophical discussion by contrasting the notions of 'human consciousness' and 'self-consciousness'. Typically, in thinking about personal identity, philosophers have tended to focus on the notion of self-consciousness. In doing so, they have followed John Locke, who as we saw in Chapter 4 spoke about the person being able to 'consider itself as itself'. There are some very good reasons for taking this view of what it is for humans to be persons. For instance, as far as we know, the ability to self-reflect is uniquely human. Self-consciousness is the ability to reflect on our conscious states. In order for this to be the ability that marks us out as human beings, it has to be consciousness over time. In other words, it is hard to conceive how I could be conscious only in an instant and still have the requisite *self*-consciousness. What I become conscious of, as a human being, even in an instant, is me. And I exist as a person over time. The significance of this point is that it suggests the pivotal role of memory. Hence, when memory goes it becomes difficult, it is argued as we saw in Chapter 4, to defend the claim that the person still exists, because the glue that holds together the self has gone.

One immediate problem with this argument concerns the definition of 'memory'. The point is that the glue (such as it is) is primarily *episodic* memory, which binds one episode of our lives to another. Clearly, this type of recall is affected in dementia. However, there are other types of memory, as we saw in Chapter 3.

For instance, as I mentioned, many of us have come across people with very poor recall who can nevertheless still play the piano (an implicit memory). The notion of emotional memory is also relevant. It sometimes seems that particular situations evoke emotions from many years previously. A further danger in giving such pre-eminence to recall memory lurks in the vagaries of testing. Sabat (2001) certainly gives examples of people performing poorly on tests of recall memory who, nevertheless, are able to demonstrate intact recall in many day-to-day situations.

I wish, however, to pursue a different point by highlighting the notion of human consciousness. What is human consciousness? The philosopher might well wish to insist that this question should be made more specific. Contrariwise, the breadth of the idea is useful. The notion of 'human consciousness' calls to mind everything that might be involved in human mental life. This is distinctly not, therefore, just those things that can be demonstrated by cognitive tests. Human consciousness suggests an openness to human relationships. Our emotions or affective states are inherently part of human consciousness. Similarly, it must involve aesthetic experience. In other words, the notion of human consciousness brings in Post's emotional, relational and aesthetic aspects of personhood.

The concept of human consciousness also gestures at shared aspects of our mental life. Jung's idea of a 'collective unconscious' comes to mind. Apart from the anthropological work that can show unities across cultures and times, there is the more mundane experience of becoming aware of (or becoming conscious of) an atmosphere in a room. This becomes highly salient if we are concerned about the emotional tone used to deal with people with dementia. But it is also important as a way of showing how our mental life is not confined to our skulls. Consider, as a further example, the way in which music communicates meanings that can be shared between people. This seems some way away from self-consciousness; thus, human consciousness expands the field of the mental.

We could, after all, talk of human self-consciousness, but my point is that the idea of *self*-consciousness, whilst interesting, is too inward-looking. In fact, the notion of the self, at least as discussed in social constructionist writings, is multifaceted. If our conceptions of the self allow that it is constructed and maintained by others, then self-consciousness should not merely relate to memory or any other cognitive function. Instead, the self is in the world and engaging with others, it is not a matter of memory. Human consciousness, then, broadly conceived, reaches out to the world and to the shared spaces in which we interact and inter-relate as human beings-in-the-world.

The intentionality and externality of mind

In considering human mental life, an important aspect of mind to consider is intentionality. As we saw in Chapter 3, certain mental states are said to be intentional in the sense that they are always *about* or *of* something: I think *of* something; my memories are memories *of* or *about* things or people. Not all mental states show this property: pain is not about something, it just is pain. What is the further significance of these states?

Intentionality shows how an aspect of mental life points beyond itself. Although the arguments are complicated, as we saw in Chapter 3, the notion of intentionality can be used to support the idea of the externalism of mind (McCulloch 2003; McGinn 1989), which I shall develop a little further here. According to externalism, 'the world enters constitutively into the individuation of states of mind' (McGinn 1989, p.9). That is to say, to have a mental state, for instance to be thinking of a tree, requires that there are things such as trees in the world. For the thought to be the thought that it is, for it to have meaning or content, the requirement is that there are trees. Otherwise it is a thought without content, without meaning. The word 'constitutively' is important. It conveys the idea that the world is inherent to the nature of mental states, because without some item in the world, in this case trees, the thought would not be the thought that it is. The external world is *constitutive* of the mental state.

As we saw in Chapter 3, the externalist account of mind suggests that the mind is not in the head. In a very real sense, we can share our thoughts: 'the walls of the mind seem...built to be breached by other substances; the mind is only too willing to share its domicile with other substances (it keeps the front door always open)' (McGinn 1989, p.22). According to externalism, different minds can reach out and embrace the same objects. Indeed, we have to have this ability in order to communicate, in order to share the same meanings. Similarly, our minds can embrace each other. We can know what someone else is thinking. Not by some sort of mystical inner process, however, but partly by the everyday observations of outward behaviour, as well as by something which does seem more mysterious, namely that we do in fact share the same public spaces in which our mental lives meet. It is the external world, in which people act and interact, that allows meaning to be conveyed. As McCulloch (2003, p.105) says: 'Doings and sayings are the primary bearers of content.'

But, of course, 'doings and sayings' are out there in the world. Much of our mental life, therefore, goes on in external space, in which our minds must engage with objects and with each other. This engagement will not always be unproblematic; it will sometimes require careful interpretation. The need for interpretation is not solely a feature of interaction with people with dementia or other disabilities. Everyday life is full of misunderstandings and the need to reinterpret and concentrate in order to grasp fully someone else's meanings or intentions. As we have commented elsewhere:

> externalism's push outwards, whereby content becomes necessarily shared, or at least shareable, makes sense of the attitude towards people with dementia according to which, however muddled their language, it might still be possible to hear their meaning through genuine attempts to engage with them phenomenologically. (Hughes *et al.* 2006, p.18)

Indeed, especially as dementia worsens, it becomes necessary to work harder in order to interpret the person's meaning. But the person with dementia retains the ability to convey meaning

(Sabat and Harré 1994), even if what is required from us is a greater effort at meaning-making (Widdershoven and Berghmans 2006).

Being minded and being a person

The move from talk of minds to talk of persons should not be made as if it were straightforward. There is clearly much more to being a person. But the externality of mind encourages us to think of personhood in a different way. Persons are minded in this particular way such that it is constitutive of them that they interact in certain ways in public space. At least, in principle human persons have this potential. Part of what it is to be a human person is precisely to have this potential to interact meaningfully. Certain illnesses, at any stage of life, are tragic inasmuch as, and to the extent that, they destroy this potential. The humane response, however, should be to nurture the possibility of such potential.

But being a person is not just to be minded. It is also to be a physical presence. It is also to participate, in one way or another (or at least to have the potential for such participation), in the world. Moreover, it is to be situated in a personal, familial, social, cultural and historical narrative. The ways in which we are situated as persons cannot be circumscribed. Our standing as situated embodied agents immediately entails that a hypercognitive description of personhood must be hopelessly inadequate if it is intended as a description of our being in the world (Hughes 2011a). We act and interact in the world in all sorts of physical ways, but (as we saw in Chapter 3) some of these physical interactions are manifestations of our mindedness. In this sense we are 'body-subjects', as Merleau-Ponty might have said. But our mindedness is also shared and the potential to share meanings, intentions, thoughts, memories and suchlike, is inherent to our standing as beings of this kind. This also entails that we are partly constituted by the narratives that we take part in, create and co-create (Baldwin and Estey-Burtt 2013).

Beyond hypercognitivism, therefore, is the world. It is a world of relationships, of emotions, of sensations, of bodily encounters, of aesthetic experience, of shared meanings, of shared and disputed values. The person is not just a disconnected atom moving through this world. The world itself in part constitutes the person. It invades our minds and shapes our understanding. Given this complexity and the sensitivity required to comprehend all of the fragile nuances of the world of persons, what will be required in health and social care is tremendous openness to the possibilities of and for the person. In particular, at the end of life, where the person's physical grip on life is tentative, and more especially where the person's mental abilities are also compromised, practitioners need to adopt a stance of great care, which will entail a broad perspective and a good deal of delicacy in their dealings with the Other.

Conclusion: Emotional, relational and aesthetic persons

This philosophical discussion shows how the notion that we are quintessentially cognitive is too facile. We are emotional and relational beings and we interact and inter-relate at an emotional level. This is not to imply a statement of empirical fact. It follows, at a conceptual level, from our being persons of this sort. When we start to describe how it is that we are minded, what it is for us to have this potential, it turns out that the concept of mind (according to externalism) is world-involving. And it involves our bodies and our interactions too.

Our situatedness as persons also entails that, to be the persons we are, we have certain sorts of relationship. Again, this can seem like an empirical point: as it happens we co-construct this particular narrative. But it is also a conceptual point. For, our meanings and our thoughts and even our memories must, in principle at least, be shareable if they are to have content. Our mindedness entails a reaching out into the world.

Part of what we share is an appreciation of the world. People with even severe dementia can respond to a soothing environment: they have aesthetic sense. I shall discuss this further in the final chapters of this book. But the potential to have this sort of appreciation, inasmuch as it is a feature of a shared sensibility, is again a demonstration of the ways in which we are minded thus. Of course, logically and empirically, we could have a different sort of sensibility, but being minded thus entails the potential to share aesthetic experiences. That this is still possible in severe dementia is a matter of empirical fact, but the philosophical discussion at least shows that there is no contradiction involved in this possibility. Moreover, uncovering the conceptually complex ways in which the mind reaches out to the world should show us the correct ways to respond to people with dementia.

Not only should it persuade us that people with severe dementia should be treated with respect, because of their persisting nature as situated embodied agents, but it should also teach us that understanding the person requires an understanding of narrative and relationships, so that decisions on the person's behalf must – as we have seen in the previous three chapters – take a broad view of what might be best. Finally, it should underscore the desire to enhance personhood in severe dementia by attention, as Stephen Post (2000) suggested, to the emotional, relational and aesthetic possibilities that characterize our standing as beings of this sort. We end where we began: with an ardent desire for good quality palliative care for people with severe dementia, supported by and supportive of a broad view of personhood, way beyond hypercognitivism.

CHAPTER 10

Understanding the Language of Distress

Introduction

I turn in this chapter to a particular clinical problem, which falls within the sphere of palliative care for people with dementia. The clinical problem is that people with severe dementia increasingly lose the ability to speak. So they cannot tell us if they are in pain. There are reasons for believing that significant numbers of people with severe dementia might be in pain and some research to suggest that many of these people are not being appropriately treated. Now, it may be that the proportion of people with severe dementia who are in pain is lower than the research suggests. For example, although there are studies suggesting that pain is commonly experienced in between 30 and 60 per cent of older people including those with dementia, in a pilot study we conducted of 79 people with severe dementia only 12 (or 16%) appeared to have pain (Jordan *et al.* 2012). There are also theoretical reasons to believe that the perception of pain might be changed by dementia. None the less, even if only 16 per cent of people with severe dementia have pain, that they cannot communicate this (at least not by speech) is a great concern. One bad way to settle the concern would be to treat them all with painkillers, but not only might this not work, it might also induce side effects. Still, there is at least one influential paper in which this has been done to good effect in that it decreased measures of both pain and agitation (Husebo *et al.* 2011). So there is a real clinical problem: how do we know whether a person is in pain if he or she cannot tell us?

This immediately suggests a philosophical problem to do with epistemology, which is the study of knowledge itself: thus, how do we *know* the person is in pain? This is a question, for instance, that the philosopher Wittgenstein, whom we have already met in several chapters, asked in *The Blue Book* (Wittgenstein 1958) and in the *Philosophical Investigations* (Wittgenstein 1968), where he contrasts knowing what it is in my *own* case to be in pain with knowing that someone else is in pain. Hence, his interlocutor says: 'I can only *believe* that someone else is in pain, but I *know* it if I am.' Wittgenstein appears to be dismissive of this attitude and concludes the paragraph by saying: 'Just try – in a real case – to doubt someone else's fear or pain' (Wittgenstein 1968, §303).

In this chapter I do not propose to follow the epistemological enquiry. Instead, I am interested in the nature of clinical judgement – in this case the judgement that someone is in pain – but quite generally the basis for judgements about diagnosis or treatment. It might be that Wittgenstein's dismissive attitude is important not because of what it tells us about the difference between knowledge and belief, but because of what it tells us about judgement as such – and this is important in all sorts of ways in clinical practice.

Pain behaviour

To return to the assessment of pain in severe dementia, one perfectly reasonable way to move forward would seem to be (at least at first blush) to identify pain behaviours in a formalized way. People have done this to derive objective measures of pain. One such instrument to measure pain is PAINAD, which was derived from a much larger observation scale with good reliability and validity. For the purposes of making the more philosophical points I wish to pursue I shall focus on PAINAD only because it is the instrument with which I am most familiar (Jordan *et al.* 2011). PAINAD looks at five domains and a person can be given a score from 0 to 2 for each domain, so that the score is out of 10. The domains are: breathing, negative vocalization, facial expression, body language and consolability. To take facial expression: smiling or a neutral expression would score zero; looking sad, frightened or frowning would lead to a score of one; whilst facial grimacing would give a score of two. There are statistical reasons to think that an overall score of two or more would suggest the probability of pain (Zwakhalen, van der Steen and Najim 2012).

All of this might seem to be straightforwardly sensible. We simply have to observe a person with severe dementia using PAINAD. If the person scored 4 or 5 we might decide to give them paracetamol; if they score 8 or 9, we might give them stronger analgesia, perhaps opioids. The difficulty for this approach, however, is that there is no behaviour that is specific for pain (Jordan, Regnard and Hughes 2007). In our study, for instance, people made 'negative vocalizations' and grimaces both because they were being lifted into a bath and they had arthritic joints (and so were deemed to be in pain) and because someone was stealing their dinner (which is upsetting but not painful)! This showed up in our statistical analysis of PAINAD (Jordan *et al.* 2011): it had a sensitivity of 92 per cent, meaning that it was very good at picking up people who were in pain; its specificity, however, was only 61 per cent, meaning that it also picked up a variety of behaviours – which scored as if they represented pain – but were not caused by pain. Instead, they were caused by things such as another resident trying to steal the person's dinner. Not all the so-called false positives were attributable to trivial matters (although having someone fiddle with your food whilst you are trying to eat is bad enough); some people were sad, anxious, fearful or possibly hallucinating.

Given this lack of correlation between so-called pain behaviours and pain, it seems more sensible to use a broader category than pain. Hence, Claud Regnard and colleagues designed an observational tool called DisDAT, which is intended to pick up distress (Regnard *et al.* 2007). The important thing is to pick up distress as the umbrella state and then to determine its cause. One cause might be pain, but other causes of distress might be hallucinations, or anxiety provoked by a lack of understanding of the situation, and so on. DisDAT makes no presumptions about the cause of distress. Just as, however, there is no specific behaviour that is unique to pain, so too there is no unique behaviour to suggest distress. Another important feature of DisDAT, therefore, is that there are no prescribed behaviours that have to be looked for. Instead, the carer who knows the person well has to decide which behaviours suggest the person is content and which suggest distress. Hence, each individual will have a *unique* list of behaviours suggesting either contentedness or distress. DisDAT generates individualized, unique measures of distress, which can then encourage thought about the causes of this particular distress. In our study, 79 people generated 129 different behaviours of distress; 72 of these were unique to an individual (Jordan *et al.* 2012). A *prescribed* list of distress behaviour (as in PAINAD and most other pain observation tools) might well include common signs, such as frowns or shouting, but would be unlikely to include items such as 'leans back when walking', 'shuffles in chair', 'rolls up trouser legs' and so forth. These were amongst many of the distress behaviours we found and were able to document as individual for individual people using DisDAT. If this much seems practically very sensible, there remains a more philosophical question about clinical judgement.

In talking about PAINAD we have said that some people were false positives: they scored as if they were in pain, but they were not in pain. The philosophical question concerns the justification for us *ever* making the clinical judgement that someone was or was not in pain. On what might such a judgement be based? And remember Wittgenstein: 'Just try – in a real case – to doubt someone else's fear or pain' (Wittgenstein 1968, §303). But now note that Wittgenstein was not just talking about 'pain' but also 'fear', which is another manifestation of distress. In fact, the questions that can be raised about pain can also be raised about distress: what sanctions us determining that in this case of rolling up one's trouser leg one is distressed, whereas in some other case one is simply having a joke? How are these judgements made, bearing in mind that much (i.e. treatment or lack of treatment) might hang on such a judgement?

There is a need to understand (what has been called) the language of distress. Part of the thinking behind DisDAT is that carers close to the person will have a better grasp of this language for the individual. It seems worthwhile to keep the notion of a language of distress in mind.

The tacit component of clinical judgements

One possibility is simply that we do not name the observations that go to make up the judgement that someone is in pain or distressed. In our study, for instance, the judgement that someone really was in pain was based not only on observation using the pain scale, but also on the person's history (derived from their notes and from nurses, carers and relatives) and on examination. Deciding that someone was in pain, therefore, as in the earlier example of bathing, depended on putting together various bits of information: not only did the person grimace, not only were the joints clearly arthritic, not only was there a history over many years of joint pain, but actual movement of the joints also produced the same sort of grimace. Perhaps in every case there are other bits of information that go together to show that the person is in pain or distressed. Perhaps at times these really are 'read' so intuitively by carers that they would find it difficult to enunciate them. Perhaps it is not just that the trouser leg goes up, but that there are also other subtle signs that go with this and are hardly noticed at a conscious level – a slight change in the vocalizations, or a slight change in the facial expression – all indicating distress. Or, perhaps carers learn things historically. Perhaps there was a time in the past when something clearly distressing happened and the trouser leg went up. Through a type of conditioning, based on closeness and intimacy, the carers have learned that this behaviour betokens distress.

If pursued, this thought would suggest that all intuition is based on observation, that with enough observations, even silent ones, it would be possible to make the judgement, whether this was a judgement about pain, distress, or some other diagnosis or treatment. In the extreme, all of this could be done by a computer and clinical acumen (or any other acumen involving complex judgements, such as business acumen) would be out of the window.

At this point, however, we can appeal to an argument from Wittgenstein to suggest that there is something about these sorts of judgement that cannot be pinned down in terms of factual observations. Thornton (2007, p.222), in his *Essential Philosophy of Psychiatry*, puts it thus: 'Even when a form of judgement can be codified as the application of a principle or rule, the application of the rule still depends on an element of uncodified skill.' This is, in a nutshell, an interpretation of the rule-following argument from Wittgenstein's *Philosophical Investigations*. I shall try to summarize this argument (more or less faithfully) in terms of clinical judgements about pain or distress.

Suppose I say to a new member of staff (Sam) that the way to determine whether a person with dementia is distressed is to observe features in the following series: O^1, O^2, O^3...and so on, where O^1 is facial frowning, O^2 is negative vocalizations, O^3 is agitated breathing and so on. How will I know when Sam has got it and knows what else might count as behaviour signifying distress? Perhaps Sam immediately spots that O^4 is crying, so that someone who cries is distressed. (Of course, a person could simulate distress by crocodile tears, but we are presuming this is not the case in order to make the series of observations, O^1, O^2, O^3 etc., more like the mathematical series that Wittgenstein considers in his writing.) Can we now say that Sam has got the hang of it? In sceptical vein, a question can always be raised about this type of learning, because it is always possible that Sam might go wrong. Perhaps he will not notice that O^{15}, pulling up the trouser leg, is also a member of the series and thus signifies distress too. The difficulty is that the rule that links a particular observation to distress always requires an interpretation; so that interpretation would also always need to be spelt out.

We can put the point in terms of language and meaning. Much of the rule-following argument in *Philosophical Investigations* considers how we can grasp the whole use of a word in a flash and be certain that we shall always use the word correctly. Well, let us take the '*language* of distress' quite seriously. How do we know when Sam has mastered it? One possibility is that we might point to Sam's understanding as an internal mental process. But we would then have to determine criteria of correctness (i.e. the normative grounds) for the mental process. Perhaps Sam has simply learnt some of the words by rote, but does not really understand the language. At each point, the sceptic can make the challenge that the connexion from word to meaning might go wrong. Rules seeming to link words and states need interpretation. A particular observation, rolling up the trouser leg, might or might not be thought part of the language of distress. Furthermore, if this is part of the language of distress, almost anything might be.

The relevant paragraph in *Philosophical Investigations* is §201:

> This was our paradox: no course of action could be determined by a rule, because every course of action can be made out to accord with the rule. The answer was: if everything can be made out to accord with the rule, then it can also be made out to conflict with it. And so there would be neither accord nor conflict here. (Wittgenstein 1968)

Distress might be signified by anything, so it is almost as if there can be no rule, and yet some things are distress and some things are not, which is rule-like. Wittgenstein continues by pointing out how we are inclined to seek interpretations – to interpret this particular behaviour as showing distress – but the interpretation requires some form of justification, which is itself an interpretation. To maintain the surety of our decisions about distress, we need the further interpretation to be effected in a rule-like manner. But this starts to sound like an infinite regress of interpretations, which suggests that a mistake has occurred. According to Wittgenstein, it is not that Sam must grasp a rule linking a particular behaviour to the language of distress and then make an interpretation that O^{10}, O^{11} and O^{12} are also instances of behaviour requiring the same rule to come into play; and another interpretation that the same rule *has* come into play; and so on. Wittgenstein concludes §201: 'What this shews is that there is a way of grasping a rule which is *not* an *interpretation*, but which is exhibited in what we call "obeying the rule" and "going against it" in actual cases' (Wittgenstein 1968).

In the following paragraph he says that 'obeying a rule' is a practice (§202). It is also like obeying an order (§206). We are trained to react in particular ways. Learning the language of distress is similar. It is rule-like in that some things amount to distress and others do not. And it may require some form of interpretation. But this is not because just anything can be distress. Judgements are made in accordance with patterns of practice. In a land where we are strangers (perhaps the land of severe dementia), according to Wittgenstein (1968), 'The common behaviour of mankind is the system of reference by means of which we interpret an unknown language' (§206). We can come to understand people in a strange land – and intuitive carers come to understand people with severe dementia – but in order to achieve this there must be – as a tacit or unspoken background – shared responses onto which interpretations can hook, without the necessity for further interpretations.

In *On Certainty* Wittgenstein says:

> Giving grounds…justifying the evidence, comes to an end; – but the end is not certain propositions' striking us immediately as true, i.e. it is not a kind of *seeing* on our part; it is our *acting*, which lies at the bottom of the language-game. (Wittgenstein 1969, §204)

The justification for Sam saying that someone is in distress comes from a type of practical know-how. It is not a matter of applying a rule in the sense that the truth conditions for the correct application of the rule can be codified. It is that certain actions on Sam's part will work; some interpretations will be correct and others incorrect, not because we can read this from some other definitive source, but because they are shown to be salient.

Thornton comments on the passage from *On Certainty* as follows:

> Wittgenstein's discussion thus inverts the normal order of priority of explicit and tacit knowledge. Even in the case of judgements

for which a universal principle can be written down, the ability to apply the principle depends on some basic shared practical responses to it. (2007, p.225)

In the *Oxford Textbook of Philosophy and Psychiatry*, the point is made as follows:

> Whenever an activity is rule governed it will rest on a basis of tacit knowledge or know-how. This will apply at all levels of practicality or theoreticity: from correctly applying a mathematical formalism or deducing a result, to the rule governed classification and recognition of signs and symptoms in medical diagnosis. All will depend upon implicit knowledge of how to go on. Any attempt to express this knowledge will itself depend on implicit knowledge left unexpressed. (Fulford, Thornton and Graham 2006, p.402)

Training Sam to understand the language of distress may involve all sorts of explanation – about how to approach people, signs to look out for, things to avoid – but, however much this sort of thing might be laid out for Sam (or codified), he has to have a background knowledge that allows him to make sense of the behaviours he comes across. (This is perhaps what Hans-Georg Gadamer (1900–2002), a German philosopher who worked in the continental tradition known as hermeneutics, meant when he spoke of the notion of *pre-understanding*.) At some point Sam's knowledge has to be tacit: knowledge that gets the whole thing started, which is presupposed in the learning and understanding of any language. It is the unspoken understanding that comes before anything else. Along similar lines, Wittgenstein says, 'What has to be accepted, the given, is – so one could say – *forms of life*' (1968, p.226). The background form of life – I have also already mentioned *patterns of practice* – is the basis upon which Sam's understanding of the language of distress is derived.

Tacit knowledge

The idea of 'tacit knowledge' derives from the work of Michael Polanyi (1891–1976). Of Hungarian Jewish extraction, he became Professor of Physical Chemistry at the University of Manchester from 1933 to 1948 and then, reflecting his increasing interest in social science and philosophy, Professor of Social Sciences from 1948 to 1958. He originally trained in Budapest in medicine and the physical sciences. His most famous work was *Personal Knowledge* (Polanyi 1958). In its Preface he starts by saying that 'personal knowledge' might seem like a contradiction, but this impression is removed 'by modifying the conception of knowing' (p. vii). He continues:

> I regard knowing as an active comprehension of the things known, an action that requires skill. Skilful knowing and doing is performed by subordinating a set of particulars, as clues or tools, to the shaping of a skilful achievement, whether practical or theoretical. (Polanyi 1958, p.vii)

Polanyi takes it that the scientist participates personally, by exercising skill, in the shaping of his scientific knowledge. He asserts: 'the aim of a skilful performance is achieved by the observance of a set of rules which are not known as such to the person following them' (p.49). Amusingly, he provides a scientific analysis of how to ride a bike and then asks: 'But does this tell us exactly how to ride a bicycle?'. He replies:

> No. You obviously cannot adjust the curvature of your bicycle's path in proportion to the ratio of your unbalance over the square of your speed; and if you could you would fall off the machine, for there are a number of other factors to be taken into account in practice which are left out in the formulation of this rule. Rules of art can be useful, but they do not determine the practice of an art; they are maxims, which can serve as a guide to an art only if they can be integrated into the practical knowledge of the art. (Polanyi 1958, p.50)

He makes great play of the importance of apprenticeship, by which means 'the apprentice unconsciously picks up the rules of the art, including those which are not explicitly known to the master himself' (p.53). He goes on to say that what he has said of skills can also be said of connoisseurship. 'The medical diagnostician's skill is as much an art of doing as it is an art of knowing'. He continues:

'Unless a doctor can recognize certain symptoms…there is no use in his reading the description of syndromes of which this symptom forms part' (p.54).

The student doctor will only learn to recognize the symptom by repeated exposure to it and authoritative teaching. Where this sort of connoisseurship exists in science, says Polanyi, 'we may assume that it persists only because it has not been possible to replace it by a measurable grading' (1958, p.55). Hence, he asserts, 'the art of knowing has remained unspecifiable at the very heart of science'.

A little later Polanyi discusses the pre-suppositions of science and suggests that these are assimilated by learning to speak the appropriate language. Remember the language of distress and the difficulty we have if we try to formulate or codify the meanings of such a language. The Wittgensteinian analysis suggested that what we learn is a practice: under the language game is a form of life, a way of reacting automatically (as if to an order), where explanations and interpretations must come to an end if there is to be a justification for our judgements within the language. Polanyi makes similar claims and I shall quote him at length:

> think of any interpretative framework and particularly of the formalism of the exact sciences. I am not speaking of the specific assertions which fill the textbooks, but of the suppositions which underlie the method by which these assertions are arrived at. We assimilate most of these pre-suppositions by learning to speak of things in a certain language…
>
> The curious thing is that we have no clear knowledge of what our pre-suppositions are and when we try to formulate them they appear quite unconvincing… I suggest now that the supposed pre-suppositions of science are so futile because the actual foundations of our scientific beliefs cannot be asserted at all. When we accept a certain set of pre-suppositions and use them as our interpretative framework, we may be said to dwell in them as we do in our own body. Their uncritical acceptance for the time being consists in a process of assimilation by which we identify ourselves with them. They are not asserted and cannot be asserted, for assertion can be made only *within* a framework with which we have identified

ourselves for the time being; as they are themselves our ultimate framework, they are essentially inarticulable. (1958, pp.59–60)

Back to clinical judgement

So can the basis of clinical judgements, that the person is distressed or in pain, ever be made explicit or codified? And if a judgement cannot be codified is this because it is 'essentially inarticulable'? In other words, is tacit knowledge tacit because it is ineffable? Or is it tacit merely because its codification would be difficult, because it would be too complex (i.e. practically impossible but not impossible in principle)?

We have already seen some indicative evidence that the code is practically difficult to pin down. The notion of distress seems to be open-ended. In this way it is like the concept of 'game', which Wittgenstein discusses. According to Luntley,

> mastery of the concept consists in the ability to see similarities between games, but without those similarities being capable of explicit articulation. That means that the seeing of the similarities is basic, it is not driven by an underlying classification. (2002, p.10)

If recognizing pain or distress is akin to recognizing that something falls under the concept of 'game', similar things can be said: when we realize that Mr Smith is in pain it's because we have seen a similarity. The more striking the similarity, which is also seen in a context so that the judgement is situated, the more confident we are that the person is in pain. But the situation is complex in a number of ways, because of the variability between individuals and the open-ended nature of the concepts that are being used. There is the person with dementia, a particular environmental setting and a variety of possible behaviours with a variety of possible interpretations. In discussing clinical judgements, Luntley states:

> Expertise involves judging from amongst a repertoire of interventions on particular elements whose complex interactions with one another produce the gross behaviour in which the doctor is interested. Given the complexity of the system, there is and can be no general rule... It requires judgement and

judgement…cannot be analysed in terms of rule-following. The technician following the rule-book has no scope for judgement, no capacity to respond to the particularities of the present case. The technician's response is prescribed by the rule… The expert does not turn to the rule book, they turn to the particularities of the case and make a judgement… (2002, p.11)

But, according to Luntley, the distinctive thing here is the character of the 'attentional skills' that the expert brings into play and from which patterned responses (clinical judgements) emerge. It is not that there are prior 'articulated rules'.

The concept of attention involves the idea of judgement, for attention is purposive and requires a capacity for judgement in monitoring and directing perception. Judgement is not something that only kicks in when the explicit rules and techniques are exhausted. Judgement has a role to play at the most basic level of concept mastery. (2002, p.5)

On Luntley's model, 'the classification is driven by the seeing; the attention already involves judgement and the pattern of the classification emerges from the attending, not the other way around' (p.5).

Once again, it is a practice that seems to be basic. Learning to discern distress or pain is a matter of mastering the sort of 'attentional skills' of which Luntley speaks. But these skills already involve judgements and the sort of personal commitment of which Polanyi spoke. For what has to be acquired is like a language, with which the person must become familiar. Hence, although the language will be rule-like, at root it will be a case of understanding a form of life, or patterns of behaviour, which will at some level be understood without explanation. As Wittgenstein says, 'If language is to be a means of communication there must be agreement not only in definitions but also (queer as this may sound) in judgments' (1968, §242).

There are fundamental shared responses that cannot be further interpreted because they provide the 'ultimate framework' that is 'essentially inarticulable'.

Conclusion

The lesson in connection with the assessment of pain or distress in people with severe dementia is that we cannot get away from the importance of expert judgements, perhaps made by skilled professionals, or perhaps made by those close to the person who are expert in the individual's language of distress. Such judgements are basic, involving the sort of 'attentional skills' of which Luntley spoke, and they inform or underpin the classification or codification of pain or distress. Thus, the philosophy supports the use of DISDAT, where someone with appropriate expertise, or connoisseurship (to use Polanyi's expression), makes judgements on an individual basis about the signs of contentedness or distress. Meanwhile, if prescriptive observational tools such as PAINAD are going to be used, they too must only be used with expertise and judgement.

CHAPTER 11

Ethics, Patterns, Causes and Pathways

In Pursuit of Good Palliative Care

Introduction

If all clinical practice is, at one and the same time, ethical by nature, then it seems right that we should devote some attention specifically to ethical issues in connection with palliative care for people with dementia. Much has been written about ethics and the end of life (e.g. Berlinger, Jennings and Wolf, 2013); in addition, a fair amount has been written about ethical issues in connection with dementia (e.g. Hughes and Baldwin 2006). But in this chapter I wish to bring some of the relevant issues together by considering the thorny considerations that arise in connection with withholding and withdrawing treatment. In the second section, I shall briefly discuss the notion of patterns of practice and the extent to which this notion might be helpful in terms of conceptualizing the ethical nature of practice in general, but here with respect to palliative care. I shall then move on, in the third section, to highlight a recent consensus statement regarding palliative care in dementia. The thing to note will be that, although the consensus statement is about clinical treatment in general, much of it relates very directly to ethical issues. Finally, but pursuing the point that practice and ethics are inextricably linked, I shall say something briefly about models and their use in dementia, as well as care pathways, given that the use of care pathways has become common, but also problematic.

Withholding and withdrawing treatment

In this section I wish to highlight some of the empirical evidence around withholding and withdrawing treatment in the context of palliative care for people with dementia. As readers will know, for several years now there has been a movement in favour of palliative care for people with dementia. The pioneer of this movement has been Ladislav Volicer (Volicer and Hurley 1998).

In 1990, Volicer published a paper with Fabiszewski which helped to encourage the idea that conservative management might be as good as active medical treatment for people with fevers who had Alzheimer's disease (Fabiszewski, Volicer and Volicer 1990). His further publications have pursued this point. The emphasis on palliative care rather than more intrusive treatments has subsequently been pursued by several other groups. Susan Mitchell and her colleagues have emphasized that advanced dementia is a terminal condition. In which case, palliative care seems the logical response. In a study that Mitchell *et al.* (2009) performed amongst nursing home residents with dementia, over the course of 18 months 54.8 per cent of the population had died. Roughly 40 per cent experienced distress caused by either dyspnoea or pain, and in their last three months over 40 per cent had burdensome interventions.

Table 11.1 Morbidity and mortality in people with advanced dementia in care homes

Condition	Probability (%)	Adjusted 6-month mortality (%)
Pneumonia	41.1	46.7
Fever	52.6	44.5
Eating problems	85.8	38.6

Source: Mitchell *et al.* 2009

As Table 11.1 shows, the study found that the probability of pneumonia was 41.1 per cent and the six-month mortality rate from pneumonia was 46.7 per cent.

Another group, in America, led by Greg Sachs and Jo Shega, has shown what can be achieved by pursuing a community-focused palliative approach (Shega *et al.* 2003). The list below records the elements of their programme. It involved a focus on:

- physical and psychological symptoms

- advance care planning

- education about disease

- connections to community resources

- co-ordination of care with an interdisciplinary team lead by a clinical nurse specialist

- patient-family centred care

- use of hospice services for end-stage patients.

Their population had a mean age of 82 years, were 75 per cent female and 82 per cent African-American. They were able to have an effect on the use of medication; to identify non-cancer pain (a third of the participants described having pain 'now' and half of the participants said that they experienced pain on a daily basis); to support the caregivers' experience; to provide an assessment of symptoms (e.g. pain, memory problems, behavioural problems, changes in mood, functional dependency, gait impairment); and to encourage hospice enrolment (Shega and Sachs 2010).

In the UK, meanwhile, Liz Sampson, in a retrospective case note study (Sampson *et al.* 2006) showed that people with dementia admitted to acute hospitals, despite their high mortality (which should indicate the appropriateness of a palliative approach), nevertheless experienced painful investigations and procedures, such as arterial blood gas sampling. In a more recent UK hospital study, Sampson's group showed that 24 per cent of those with severe cognitive impairment died during their acute admission, with an adjusted mortality risk of just over four. The risk of dying increased as cognitive impairment worsened. The paper concluded:

> We cannot judge from our data whether these admissions were necessary, but the high short-term mortality risk in people with

dementia suggests that this intervention did not prolong life for a meaningful length of time. Individuals may have received better-quality care in a familiar environment if more support was available in the community. (Sampson *et al.* 2009)

In the Netherlands there has been a very strong research programme over several years looking at palliative care for people with dementia. Jenny van der Steen's work with colleagues has helped to demonstrate that pneumonia is not always the old person's friend (van der Steen *et al.* 2002a). There can be considerable distress. It makes sense to think of antibiotic treatment not solely as a curative treatment, but also as a potential palliative measure. In further research van der Steen and colleagues (van der Steen *et al.* 2002b) have shown that quite nuanced judgements are made by clinicians when they are faced with someone suffering from fever and likely infection in the context of end-stage dementia. In some cases antibiotics will be used with curative intent, presumably because the physician feels that the pneumonia is not 'terminal', so that if treatment were to be withheld the person would simply be condemned to a longer period of suffering after which he or she would probably recover in any case. On the other hand, physicians sometimes say that they are using antibiotics purely as a palliative measure. For instance, there is some evidence that antibiotics can make secretions less thick and thereby ease symptoms. Finally, there is a proportion of patients in which antibiotic treatment is withheld where the belief is that the illness is so severe that death seems inevitable.

To summarize quite broadly, empirical research has helped to establish *at least* two things. First, that people with severe dementia require active treatment because they carry a significant burden of symptoms not least of which are pain and distress, but, second, that the approach should be palliative. On the other hand, we need, perhaps, to take a broad view of what 'palliative' might mean. Cees Hertogh (2010) argued that palliative care, whilst aiming at the well-being of the patient, could still include the possibility of treatments that would perhaps be *life-prolonging*. On the other hand, he said, 'symptomatic care entails *a medical policy in which a life-prolonging side effect is emphatically unwanted'* (Hertogh 2010, p.277). He records that the tendency in the Netherlands, as elsewhere, is not to try to prolong life in the case of people with dementia. This seems right inasmuch as it still involves keeping the person as symptom-free as possible. The empirical evidence, such as it is (Hughes *et al.* 2007; van der Steen 2010), argues *against* the use of artificial nutrition and hydration in severe dementia, *against* the use of antibiotics for severe infection except as a means to relieve symptoms (but not necessarily with curative intent), *against* cardiopulmonary resuscitation. I shall come to the consensus statement regarding this evidence shortly. The question, meanwhile, is how this sort of approach might be justified in ethical terms.

Specifically in connection with withholding and withdrawing treatments, there is a well-established doctrine, the Doctrine of Ordinary and Extraordinary Means, which is helpful both intellectually and practically in that it can be used to discuss these difficult issues with patients, family, other informal carers and, indeed, health and social care workers. Broadly, the doctrine states that we are morally obliged to pursue ordinary investigations and treatments. But we are not morally obliged to pursue extraordinary investigations and treatment. It is important to note this wording, because it follows that extraordinary treatment is not always inappropriate. It is just that we are not *morally obliged* to pursue extraordinary treatment. But there may be other factors that encourage us to do so. The question then is, what is it that distinguishes ordinary from extraordinary as far as investigation and treatment are concerned?

Extraordinary care is regarded as anything that is unlikely to work (in other words, it could be considered futile) and is likely to be burdensome to the person and to close family. In the case of cardiopulmonary resuscitation, therefore, we have evidence that this is unlikely to work in people with severe dementia. In addition, in severe dementia, by which I mean the really terminal stages when the person is extremely physically frail, cardiopulmonary resuscitation is very likely to be burdensome in the sense that it may well cause harm or damage to the person, for instance by fracturing ribs. There is a sense in which it might be burdensome for the family, too, because it entails that the very end of the person's life is lacking in dignity and is somewhat traumatic. So we can say, in line with the Doctrine of Ordinary and Extraordinary Means, that we are not morally obliged to pursue cardiopulmonary resuscitation in someone with end-stage dementia.

To go back to the point, however, that there may be other reasons to pursue an investigation or treatment that would normally seem to be extraordinary, it could be that a decision is made to allow cardiopulmonary resuscitation on the grounds that there is some uncertainty as to whether or not the person really is in the final stages of their dementia. Some people, for instance, have very severe dementia but remain alert or mobile. It may be that the decision is that it would be too difficult not to attempt resuscitation and too upsetting for staff and family not to do so in someone who is otherwise looking physically better than might be expected given their level of dementia. Or, perhaps, it is known that the family are travelling from abroad to be with their loved one and it is felt appropriate to try to resuscitate the patient in anticipation of their return. So there may be somewhat extraordinary circumstances in which, nevertheless, extraordinary means are taken to treat and care for the person concerned.

With that specific doctrine in place, the point I now wish to suggest is that the broader understanding of our ethical decisions at the end of life can be facilitated by considering the notion of patterns of practice.

Patterns of practice

I want to suggest that the notion of patterns of practice might be helpful in two ways. First, it might provide some guidance around how, in practice, ethical decisions should be made. Second, however, I think it provides a conceptual framework for ethical decision-making. In other words, it allows us to understand the underpinning basis of our ethical decisions. In a sense, this takes us back to some of the discussion about the externality of mind in Chapters 3 and 9. In the next chapter, I discuss intentions in more detail. Suffice it to say an intention to care, in my view, is not something that only exists in the person's head. My intention to care has to be understood as involving, constitutively, certain established patterns of practice or patterns of care. I cannot say that I intended to care for someone if I have then done something incredibly callous and mean. There is a normative demand that some patterns of practice could not be reconciled with the notion of intending to care. Just to give an extreme example, we do not care for residents in nursing homes if we assault them! But there is such a thing as careful touching and careful cleansing and the intention to care is realized in the practice of caring in particular ways and not in others. Our particular patterns are established in a complex fashion reflecting everything from upbringing, to education, to social norms and laws, to religious beliefs and adherence to particular moral traditions (Hughes 2006b).

My suggestion is that our patterns of practice provide the real basis for claiming that our decisions and actions are morally justified. However, it cannot be that just *anything* is justified.

Patterns of practice must be justified in terms of their internal and external *coherence*. *Internal coherence* can be usefully judged by a casuistic process. Casuistry involves looking at individual decisions case by case, where the details of the case are paramount and where particular cases are then compared to other similar cases to try to highlight points of moral difference (Louw and Hughes 2005). In other words, if I have decided not to resuscitate this particular 75-year-old man I need to consider why last week it seemed right to resuscitate another man of the same age. As a further example of a casuistic argument, if it were obvious that a person was in the severe stages of cancer there would have to be very particular reasons to check their arterial blood gases. Why, then, would this need to be done in someone with severe dementia, bearing in mind the evidence that dementia is a terminal condition?

External coherence requires that I compare my patterns of practice with broader ethical norms. Now, in my view these are provided by considering the virtues. In other words, when we judge particular actions, we need to ask whether or not they would conform to ideas about human flourishing, where flourishing is defined in terms of the virtues. Virtue theory lies behind virtue ethics, which is the third of the main ethical theories. The other two are consequentialism and deontology. Virtue ethics, however, has been ignored for a very long time, although there has been a sustained resurgence of interest in virtue theory and virtue ethics in the last 50 years (Hursthouse 1999). In brief, virtue ethics suggests that when we judge particular actions, we need to ask whether or not they would conform to ideas about human flourishing, where this is defined in terms of the virtues. Given that the good (or flourishing) human being is not dishonest and lacking in charity, the good doctor – whilst discussing with a family the likely outcome and treatment options for a person with advanced dementia suffering a severe pneumonia – should be honest and charitable.

I wish to suggest that, at the level of clinical practice, ultimate justification sits in the background practices that make up our shared world, where this encapsulates values, personal histories, social narratives and the like. But beyond this is an appeal to something of real human significance, some idea of what it is to be a good, flourishing, human being. Some facts about the world and our way of being in the world must, in my view, be pertinent here; as Philippa Foot argued: 'the grounding of a moral argument is ultimately in facts about human life' (Foot 2001, p.24).

To summarize, when we make ethical decisions, in my view, we are often using a casuistic approach. That is, we normally act in line with how we have acted before unless there are significant differences between the previous case and the current case. These differences may be empirical and reflect biological factors; for instance, blood tests may show that the person in front of us now is in a more compromised state than the last person we saw. But there may also be psychological, social, legal and ethical factors which make the current case different from the last case. This, I think, is the way that we make our day-to-day clinical decisions, in keeping with our patterns of practice, without even realizing their ethical nature, or perhaps not reflecting on this overtly, because the practice simply fits into a well-established pattern.

But when we are challenged, or when there is a more difficult problem, it may then be that we have to question our decisions from an external standpoint. Here, I suggest, the virtues play a role in that they define for us what it is to live our human lives as best we can as flourishing human beings. There may have to be compromises. It may be that no decision seems to be a good one, but nevertheless we should try to do what the virtuous person would do, because the virtuous person would act in a way such as to do well humanly. This is almost by definition, since the virtues define what it is to do well humanly or to flourish as a human being.

The white paper

In this section I wish to highlight the important publication, again led by Jenny van der Steen, which, in a white paper produced for the European Association for Palliative Care, an attempt has been made to define optimal palliative care for older people with dementia (van der Steen *et al.* 2013). Part of the reason for doing this is to emphasize that optimal palliative care is also ethical palliative care.

The white paper defines palliative care for people with dementia. It does this by setting out 11 domains that need to be considered in providing palliative care for older people with dementia. It also defines optimal care by presenting 57 recommendations regarding practice, policy and research, which fall within the 11 domains. Each of these recommendations is supported by an explanatory text. The text is based on evidence from the literature, with 265 references, and also on a consensus study using the Delphi method with experts from across the globe. Thus, experts from across the world were approached and 72 per cent of them – 64 experts from 23 countries – evaluated the domains and the recommendations in the paper. Most of the experts came from Europe, but a significant proportion came from North America and some came from South America, Australia and New Zealand, as well as the Far and Middle

East. The white paper suggests a model that might be used to prioritize the goals of care at different stages in dementia. There are also some recommendations about research. I shall not attempt here to summarize the whole of the paper.

In the Delphi part of the study, which involved the experts being sent the domains and recommendations on two occasions, there was full and immediate consensus on eight of the domains, which were around:

- person-centred care
- communication and shared decision-making
- optimal treatment of symptoms and providing care
- setting care goals and advance planning
- continuity of care
- family care and involvement
- education of the healthcare team
- societal and ethical issues.

Full consensus was also achieved, after one revision, concerning the domain on prognostication and the recognition of dying. There was, however, only moderate consensus on two other domains: the first was to do with nutrition and dehydration, where the issue was over avoiding aggressive, burdensome or futile treatments. The second was to do with dementia stages in relation to care goals, where the applicability of the palliative care model was questioned. It should be said that in both of these domains there was still a moderate degree of consensus, it was just that there was also more divergence of views than there was for the other nine domains.

Table 11.2 Importance of domains and rating of priorities for research

Domains	Clinical importance	Research priority
Applicability of palliative care	10	4
Person-centred care, communication, shared decision-making	2	1
Setting care goals, advance planning	9	3
Continuity of care	8	7
Prognostication, recognizing dying	11	8
Avoiding overly aggressive treatment	5	5
Optimal treatment: symptoms + comfort	1	2
Psychosocial and spiritual support	7	10
Family care and involvement	3	6
Education of healthcare team	6	9
Societal and ethical issues	4	11

Source: Adapted from van der Steen *et al.* 2013

Table 11.2 shows the ranked clinical importance of the different domains and also the rank they were given in terms of research priority by the experts in the Delphi study. It is interesting to note that there was good agreement that person-centred care, communication and shared decision-making were considered important both clinically and as a research priority. Similarly, optimal treatment of symptoms and the provision of comfort were also considered to be clinically very important and important for research. But if we look at the applicability of the palliative care model, that is, the question as to whether or not it is applicable to dementia, this was not thought to be a particularly important domain clinically, although it was thought to be reasonably important as a research priority. Contrariwise, societal and ethical issues were considered to be very important clinically, but were not seen as a research priority.

Box 11.1 Domain 2: Person-centred care, communication and shared decision-making

2.1 Perceived problems in caring for a patient with dementia should be viewed from the patient's perspective, applying the concept of person-centred care.

2.2 Shared decision-making includes the patient and family caregiver as partners and is an appealing model that should be aimed for.

2.3 The healthcare team should ask for and address families' and patients' information needs on the course of the dementia trajectory, palliative care and involvement in care.

2.4 Responding to the patient's and family's specific and varying needs throughout the disease trajectory is paramount.

2.5 Current or previously expressed preferences with regard to place of care should be honoured as a principle, but best interest, safety and family caregiver burden issues should also be given weight in decisions on place of care.

2.6 Within the multidisciplinary team, patient and family issues should be discussed on a regular basis.

(Recommendations from van der Steen *et al.* 2013)

In Box 11.1 I have set out the recommendations that fall within Domain 2, to do with person-centred care, communication and shared decision-making, which was considered to be very important by the experts. The recommendations, which define optimal care, can also be regarded as essentially ethical. Some of them are more obviously ethical, for instance that we should try to take the perspective of the person with dementia, but even the stipulation that the patient and family issues should be discussed on a regular basis in the multidisciplinary team sounds like an ethical principle. In other words, it sounds like the sort of thing that we *ought* to do rather than something which it is merely accepted practice to do. This is not the place to set out all of the recommendations from the white paper, but I would certainly commend this paper to the reader.

Towards the end of the paper, a model is set out to help consider the priorities of care. It should be said, again, that there was only moderate agreement about the model, which is shown in Figure 11.1.

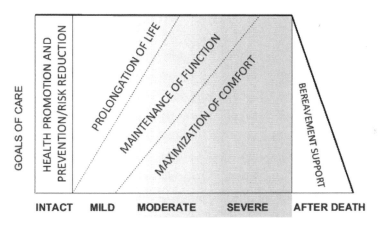

**Figure 11.1 Dementia progression and
suggested prioritizing of care goals**
Source: van der Steen *et al.* 2013

What we can see in Figure 11.1 is that, early in the course of dementia, it is suggested that the prolongation of life is an appropriate goal of care. This becomes less appropriate as dementia worsens. But even in moderate dementia it might still be an appropriate goal, albeit the maintenance of function and the maximization of comfort also become more relevant. By the time the person enters the severer stages of dementia, the model suggests that the maximization of comfort should be the main priority in terms of care. As suggested in my earlier discussion of ordinary and extraordinary means, there will, inevitably, have to be judgements about when the person is in the moderate or severe stage of their condition, and this may not always be entirely clear. And it may be, on ethical grounds, that a decision is made to provide extraordinary care for an individual despite there being no moral imperative to do so.

Models and pathways

Various models are used to understand dementia. For instance, it can be understood in a very biological way by looking at the neuropathology and the abnormal neurochemistry. This is important. But we have also seen a gradual broadening of the models used to understand dementia, just as we have similarly seen broader models emerge in other areas. So, for instance, it is common enough to hear people speak of the biopsychosocial model of disease (Engel 1980). In dementia, a big step forward – in fact it is part of what has been called the new culture of dementia care – was the work of Tom Kitwood, who talked of 'malignant social psychology' (Kitwood 1997, pp.45–49). This refers to the way in which the psychosocial environment can make things worse for the person with dementia whatever the state of his or her brain pathology. Kitwood (1997) stressed that we need to take a broader view of the person and see the extent to which relationships affect the standing of the person. There can be attitudes and actions which detract from the person's well-being, just as there can be attitudes and actions which enhance the person's well-being. Person-centred dementia care, therefore, does not deny the importance of biological care, but places greater emphasis on psychosocial care. Similar concerns to avoid 'malignant positioning' can be seen in the work of Steve Sabat (2001). Thinking in this way, we could then regard the palliative care model as either very similar to the person-centred care model, or perhaps as an enlargement of that model. It is an enlargement only in the sense that it makes more frequent and overt mention of spiritual care as well as biopsychosocial care. This is not to say that Kitwood ignored spiritual care, for indeed he did not (Baldwin and Capstick 2007). Nevertheless, whereas the biomedical model can be regarded as focusing on pathology, which leads to symptoms and signs, the biopsychosocial model broadens the perspective to include the psychosocial context. The palliative care model can be regarded as broadening the perspective further to give an holistic view. The holistic view includes the spiritual dimension, but also places a significant emphasis on the importance of the family for the person concerned. Beyond the palliative care model, we come to the supportive care model (Hughes, Lloyd-Williams and Sachs 2010).

The supportive care model can be regarded as broader still in that it allows that anything that might be helpful should be pursued. It is broad in the sense that it allows discussion of care from the time of diagnosis until beyond death, when relatives are grieving. The term 'supportive care' in itself seems to place less emphasis on death, whereas 'palliative' is often associated with death and dying. The supportive care model also does away with the dichotomies of care versus cure, or of high technology versus low technology, or of biological against social, or the dichotomy between patient-centred care and carer-centred care and, finally, the dichotomy concerning 'being with' and 'doing to' someone. In short, anything that might be helpful should be done. The questions for the supportive care model are: what needs to be done now? And how may we help? I do not wish to pursue a fuller description of the supportive care model here, because more details of supportive care for people with dementia exist elsewhere (Hughes *et al.* 2010).

Nevertheless, I do wish to raise a question about the nature of models, given that what we see in the broadening out of the focus of the models is something that seems to be both beneficial and good. It seems more likely that we will be able to help the person if we take the broadest possible view. It also seems likely that we will make the right decision (in the sense of the ethical decision) if our perspective is broad enough. But this then raises a question. If this movement of broadening out is good, where does it lead?

Well, my suggestion is that it leads to a world without models. In other words, I wish to make the point that when we meet someone, we do not normally use a model to understand the person. Of course, we can do so in particular circumstances. The meeting between two people, however, does not require the use of models. Elsewhere I have said this: 'The world without models is the world of real human encounters, where embodied subjects meet in the raw. But the world without models is also a world without science' (Hughes 2011a, p.208). This is not an anti-science point, but it is intended to situate science in its proper context, which is the context of human endeavours in which any particular scientific understanding will occupy a specific area. Health and social care professionals, therefore, first meet people as human beings and engage with them as such. For particular purposes, they may then use a specific model in an attempt to be helpful in this way or that. But the scientific understanding is embedded in the human understanding.

This takes me on to the second theme of this section, which is to consider care pathways. I shall make a similar point, namely that care pathways must not lose sight of the individual human beings with which they are concerned. A care pathway can too easily become merely numerous sheets of paper with numerous tick boxes, which have to be completed by busy staff. In the UK, there has recently been a furore over the Liverpool Care Pathway for the dying. This was successfully used and implemented within palliative care, specifically in hospices, but as its use was spread to the broader National Health Service (NHS) problems emerged. The accusations, which finally led to the Liverpool Care Pathway being withdrawn, include the suggestion that more time was spent filling in the forms than really providing good quality care. Indeed, the accusations are worse than this, namely that the care was actually deficient despite the pathway, and maybe because of it. The rights and wrongs of the use of the Liverpool Care Pathway need not detain us. But the issues will be apparent. It is for this reason that I wish to suggest the features that should underlie the ideal care pathway in reality.

Before doing so, however, I need to revisit the notion of values-based practice (mentioned in passing in Chapter 8). The 10 principles of values-based practice (VBP), as described by Fulford (2004) are shown in Box 11.2.

Box 11.2 Principles of values-based medicine ──────────

(1) *The two-feet principle*: All clinical decisions require attention to both facts and values.

(2) *The squeaky wheel principle*: Values become more noticeable when they are diverse or conflicting.

(3) *The science-driven principle*: Progress makes values more apparent.

(4) *The patient-perspective principle*: Patients should always be heard.

(5) *The multiperspective principle*: We cannot assume that the values of others are the same as our own: values are diverse.

(6) *The values-blindness principle*: Awareness of values will be encouraged by careful attention to what people say.

(7) *The values-myopia principle*: Differences are legitimate and must be taken into account.

(8) *The space of values principle*: Where values conflict, the right outcome will generally come from a process that supports the legitimately held views of others.

(9) *The how it's done principle*: It requires good communication, with negotiation concerning values.

(10) *The who decides principle*: Decisions should be made on the basis of partnership.

Adapted from Fulford 2004, p.206

Again, there is much more that could be said about values-based practice (Fulford, Peile and Carroll 2012). But, for my purposes, there are two important things to be derived. First, values-based practice, which complements evidence-based practice, recognizes in an overt way the importance of values, both when they are shared and also when they are diverse and, consequently, more likely to be disputed. Second, values-based practice suggests that communication is the way to move forward when there are conflicts of values. Values diversity, in other words, has to be negotiated in a skilful way. The values of everyone concerned must be taken into account, but the person (in this case) with dementia should be put first even if, in the given context, his or her values cannot be fully realized.

With the notion of values-based practice in place, along with the idea that models must be as broad as possible, not only to include biological, psychological and social perspectives, but also spiritual, as well as ethical and legal issues, it is then possible to set out what is involved in a care pathway.

Of course, there must be a care co-ordinator and of course there should be some advance care planning (as discussed in Chapter 7). But then we also need to have the full spectrum of components of supportive care, that is the broadest possible model, as might be indicated by the different elements in Table 11.3.

Table 11.3 Examples of components of supportive care

Biological	Psychological	Social	Spiritual	Ethical and legal
Genetics	Counselling	Lifestyle	Spiritual support	Person-centred care
Biological risk factors	Emotional support	Environmental risks (e.g. 'wandering')	Religious practices	Giving the diagnosis
Anti-dementia drugs	Cognitive stimulation	Day care	Quality of life	Decision-making
Optimizing physical treatment	Aromatherapy	Personalized budgets	Working through	Advance care planning
Pain management	Carer burden	Dementia café	Complementary therapies	Doctrine of double effect
Falls reduction	Therapeutic relationships	Suitable accommodation	Namaste care	Maintaining dignity
Nutritional support	Meaningful activities	Services for people in remote areas	'Being with' as well as 'doing to'	Issues around driving

Source: Derived from Hughes *et al.* 2010, p.100
(see also Hughes 2013b, Table 3, p.13)

The care pathway, then, represents a journey, which is made by the person with dementia, but which is usually not made alone. The person is accompanied by family and friends, but also by professionals. Together they will be entering a terrain, which involves ethical and legal, spiritual, social, psychological and biological factors. The journey will require careful navigation, as well as negotiation when values appear to be in conflict. The outcome, however, should be that the person's experience within any of these individual domains at any stage of the journey is optimal. All of this may be facilitated by tick boxes on paper or on a computer, but fundamentally the journey is the journey of *human beings engaged with each other in the raw* with all the complexities that arise in the real world.

Conclusion

In this chapter I have discussed some of the ethical and empirical issues around withholding and withdrawing treatment for people with palliative care needs and dementia. I have then considered the background patterns of practice that help us to conceptualize how we make ethical decisions. I have considered the consensus around the recommendations of the white paper concerning palliative care for people with dementia, partly in order to draw out the ethical nature of many of these recommendations. I have then, finally, suggested that we encounter each other without models and that our care pathways should be about human relationships, taking into account the breadth of such relationships and the complexity of the context in which these relationships occur, a context which involves both facts and values.

I feel I should end by saying something about assisted dying, given this is an ethically contested area. These remarks are only brief in anticipation of further remarks in the next chapter.

A refusal to contemplate the possibility of active voluntary euthanasia or physician-assisted suicide can sometimes seem callous or lacking in compassion and these are not virtues that would encourage human flourishing. But, of course, we cannot call just anything callous or lacking in compassion. The normativity that governs our use of language is embedded in our practices, which has implications for *all* our clinical judgements. Our intentions are played out in public: not just *any* behaviour is in keeping with having a good intention.

The problem is to agree, which I do not think we do in the modern world, on what it is in the background to our lives that gives significance, which (to borrow from Charles Taylor) provides 'a background of intelligibility' (Taylor 1991, p.37). Taylor also suggests that, 'I can define my identity only against the background of things that matter'. I want to suggest that the virtues, mentioned in connection with patterns of practice, are candidates for this sort of 'horizon' of significance. But others will disagree. To sanction assisted dying, however, will require that human life *in itself* (and those words are critical) is not seen as the source of flourishing, is not seen in this sense as a good, is not seen as embedded in a history, in a moral, legal and social context that involves a prohibition on killing. In the absence of such a sanction, where human life in itself *is* seen as the source of flourishing, and *is* seen in this sense as a good, then human life, even in severe dementia, remains worthy of care even if the care does not aim at prolonging life but instead accepts the concrete reality of approaching death and seeks to ease the person's death by all means possible.

I think that understanding thought and language in relation to the mind and mental phenomena tells us something about how we relate to the world. I shall say more about this in the next chapter.

We are not disconnected autonomous atoms moving in a free sea of our own wishes and inclinations, guided by our inner psychological realities. We are, on the contrary, interconnected, interdependent, social beings driven by biology, as well as by our psychology, sociology, spirituality, legal systems, history, moral dispositions, culture and so forth. In brief, we are *situated* embodied agents, where none of our actions is inconsequential. For, to quote John Donne (1572–1631),

> No man is an island, entire of itself; every man is a piece of the continent, a part of the main. If a clod be washed away by the sea, Europe is the less, as well as if a promontory were, as well as

if a manor of thy friend's or of thine own were: any man's death diminishes me, because I am involved in mankind, and therefore never send to know for whom the bell tolls; it tolls for thee. (Donne 1999, Meditation XVII)

CHAPTER 12

Intentions and Best Interests

Dying and Killing

Introduction

In this chapter I shall suggest that the correct attitude towards people with severe dementia is the palliative approach. I see the palliative approach as being at odds with any form of euthanasia approach, where this involves intentional active killing or physician-assisted suicide. In saying this I know of no grounds for suggesting that a palliative approach has ever entailed preserving life at all costs. Indeed, one of the good things about the palliative approach, in my opinion, is that it shows a realistic and appropriate acceptance of death. My personal view, in brief, is that I think there are numerous circumstances, especially in severe dementia, where we should be allowing nature to take its course and, indeed, easing the person's dying, but I could envisage it neither as my role to kill people with severe dementia nor to assist them in doing so themselves.

There are numerous arguments about voluntary euthanasia and assisted suicide. The best single volume to encapsulate arguments on both sides of the debate is, in my opinion, still Keown (1995). My own arguments are captured in a debate with Philip Graham (Graham and Hughes 2014). Rather than try to rehearse every argument here, I shall – on the basis of the situated-embodied-agent view of the person – argue three things: first, that personhood persists even into severe dementia, second, that best interests must be understood as broadly as possible, and third, that intentions are not just 'inner', but are embedded in a context. In turn, these three conclusions suggest to me three further claims that support the palliative approach in dementia. First, as persons, people with dementia cannot be morally disregarded: they deserve the same sort of care as any one else. Second, a broad view of best interests commends the holism of palliative care. Third, the judgement of an action must include reference to its intentional nature, which is shown both by context as well as by aim. It is particularly (but not solely) the third claim that counts against the type of killing that occurs in active voluntary euthanasia. For once an action is described as an act of intentional killing of the innocent, according to my lights, it should be condemned. I suspect this third claim requires acceptance of another premise, namely that life is a good, and I want to say something about this too, albeit very briefly.

Back to the SEA view

Philosophy in this country used to be very analytic or linguistic. It still is, of course, because good philosophy needs to be analytic in this sense. But it is now more open to continental influences. I do not intend to enter the debates that have raged about the merits and demerits of (so-called) analytic and continental philosophy. What I wish to do is just to highlight an important development, which is relevant to our thoughts about personhood in dementia.

The analytic tradition was hot on words and definitions and it was also very rational, maybe even intellectualist, or perhaps cognitivist. What continental philosophy and the later Wittgenstein brought in was a greater awareness of context, culture, history, narrative, public space, inter-relatedness, the body and so forth. I think that the SEA view, introduced in Chapter 4, whilst reflecting the analytic tradition of thinkers such as Locke and Parfit, brings in a whole lot more besides. It derives from numerous thinkers, but is perhaps summed up in the writings of Charles Taylor (1989), who reflects both the continental tradition and the later Wittgenstein, as well as the more analytic, linguistic school. Part of my intention in suggesting this view is also to suggest that what it is to be a person cannot be circumscribed. This view suggests that there are always further possibilities for individual human beings.

Stephen Post, the American ethicist and expert on dementia whom we encountered in Chapter 9, has written:

> Rationality is too severe a ground for moral standing, allowing (if not requiring) the disregard of many individuals who share our common humanity from the edges of decline.
>
> …
>
> Even in the advanced stage of dementia…one finds varying degrees of emotional and relational expression, remnants of personality, and even meaningful non-verbal communication (as in the reaching out for a hug). (Post 2006, p.231)

As we saw in Chapter 9, Post also argues in favour of hospice care for people with severe dementia. He does this whilst emphasizing the broader aspects of personhood – the body to be touched for instance – including the importance of the person's inevitable situatedness and, therefore, relatedness to others. More than that, the person is maintained as a person by this inter-relatedness.

Similarly, Rom Harré – in the slightly different field of social psychology – has fought a battle against what he has termed the cognitive revolution in psychology. Cognitive psychology, in broad terms, seeks to understand the mind by analogy with the computer. The mind has inputs, inner processes and representations, and outputs. Harré prefers to emphasize the social aspects of the mind. Our mental life, according to Harré, is socially embedded, in our conversations for instance. It is out there in the world, where we inter-relate, rather than stuck inside our craniums. Harré writes:

> In the restoration of personal psychology, I want to bring back the study of endeavour, conatus, striving, trying and the like. In the conditions for the use of these concepts I feel the presence of persons as agents rather than as passive passengers on a mental vehicle directed and powered by subpersonal vectors (or information-processing modules) of various kinds. (Harré 1983, p.185)

The recognition that there are aspects of the self that depend on other people led Harré, in conjunction with Steve Sabat, to consider people with dementia and the extent to which they are still semiotic subjects, that is selves that can convey meaning (Sabat and Harré 1994). In his later work, Sabat has emphasized the need to look beyond the cognitive tests of people with dementia, which can amount to what he terms 'defectology', in order to see the person's potential to interact, once given an appropriately benign social environment. This sort of social environment, devoid of what Tom Kitwood has called 'malignant social psychology' (Kitwood 1997), will itself be sustaining of the person's self. Our attitudes to people with dementia can too easily position them as impaired and second class.

> Realistic, accurate positioning would require healthy others to take into account the effects not only of the disease itself, and the afflicted person's reactions to the effects of the disease, but also the effects of the social environment on the afflicted person's behavior. (Sabat 2001, p.111)

It would be possible to continue in this way, pointing to various authors within the field of dementia care who have urged that people with dementia must be seen as persons through and through. Most famously, perhaps, Tom Kitwood (1997) encouraged the notion of person-centred care in connection with people with dementia. As this quote shows, at the core of person-centred care is the importance of relationships:

> Memory may have faded, but something of the past is known; identity remains intact, because others hold it in place; thoughts may have disappeared, but there are still interpersonal processes; feelings are expressed and meet a validating response; and if there is a spirituality, it will likely be of the kind that Buber describes, where the divine is encountered in the depth of I–Thou relating. (Kitwood 1997, p.69)

My intention now, rather than appealing any further to the authority of those who write within the context of the new culture of dementia care, is to argue the three points I raised at the beginning of this chapter: first, that personhood persists even into severe dementia, second, that best interests must be understood as broadly as possible, and third, that intentions are not just 'inner', but are embedded in a context. These arguments will lead to my claims about palliative care.

Personhood in severe dementia

I have already mentioned (in Chapter 4) the idea that personal identity, roughly speaking, depends on memory. This has led a number of commentators to suggest that in severe dementia personhood must be lost because memory is lost. One argument against this suggestion, however, is that it is too simplistic. People with dementia do occasionally say lucid things, showing that their awareness and recall are still intact, at least to a degree. There are dramatic stories, in connection with the use of anti-dementia drugs, of people who seem to have been 'lost', but who then recover and can recall what happened to them when they were inaccessible, suggesting that the self was still there all along. In the same passage quoted earlier, Post says:

> The reality is that until the very advanced and even terminal stage of dementia, the person with dementia will usually have sporadically articulated memories of deeply meaningful events and relationships ensconced in long-term memory. (Post 2006, p.231)

But even if, at some stage, all memories were lost, the SEA view of the person argues in favour of continuing personhood. As I argued in Chapter 5, the person with dementia can still demonstrate agency through gestures, vocalizations, grimaces, emotional tone and so forth. These cannot be dismissed as *mere* gestures, like the gestures of a pet animal, because they are situated in the individual's human context. They can convey meaning; they can be interpreted on the basis of prior knowledge, they can be assessed, albeit with difficulty, as suggesting human anxiety, anguish, pleasure, pain, contentedness, sadness and so on. In keeping with Post's suggestion, situated agency is not lost until the person is more or less comatose, when they are then no different from anyone else who is dying.

One thing this immediately suggests is that the requirement towards the end of the person's life in severe dementia is for him or her to have a higher level of skilled care, specialist palliative care even. We need nurses with *exceptional* skills in dementia care, because this sort of nursing is going to be difficult. I am taking it for granted that to allow someone's personhood to dissipate through lack of care would be a great wrong. The trend otherwise is to say that in these advanced stages of dementia the person might 'only' require general nursing care. But I think that, if we take the possibility of the person's situated agency seriously, we shall need specialist *dementia* palliative care. Furthermore, such a service would have to become involved with the person with dementia at an earlier stage if the staff are to build up the relationships that would allow the correct interpretations and judgements to be made.

The persistence of personhood into severe dementia, therefore, argues in favour of good quality palliative care, the type of care we should like to see for all persons suffering from chronic illnesses that cannot be cured. The evidence is that people with dementia (in a similar way to people with other non-cancer chronic conditions) are not treated in an equitable fashion as regards palliative care (Hughes, Robinson and Volicer 2005). This certainly cannot be excused on the grounds that these people do not count. The SEA view supports the idea that human beings can be persons in different ways, but persons none the less. If this is true, it undercuts those who suggest that euthanasia should be allowable for people with dementia because they are, in some sense, not persons, or lesser persons. However, it is not an argument *in itself* against active voluntary euthanasia or physician-assisted dying and, if euthanasia becomes allowable for others in society, there is no reason, on *this* ground, for not allowing it – with proper provisions – for people with dementia. The continuing personhood of people with dementia cuts away some of the grounds for killing such people, but might allow that they can be intentionally killed by their doctors on other grounds, if it is the case that their doctors are allowed to kill other people who do not have dementia.

Best interests and the SEA view

The second argument I wish to put forward on the basis of the SEA view of the person is that it suggests that best interests must be understood as broadly as possible. Especially in dementia, determining someone's best interests is always difficult. Actually, the *whole concept* is difficult. We might normally think that people should judge what is best for themselves: after all we are the ones with the best reason to have an interest in our best interests! But even this is not true. Many of us would *not* wish to claim that *we* know what is best for us; we are prone to seek advice about what this might be under specific circumstances. However, equally, most of us, I think, would not accept that any other particular individual had indubitable insight into what was best for us; not, that is, without knowing a whole lot about us, about our wishes, inclinations, desires, values, character, aspirations, etcetera. In other words, figuring out what is best entails a pretty thorough understanding of *how* we are situated as embodied agents. And, although I have a privileged position concerning how *I* am situated, this does not prevent *others* from also having a legitimate perspective on how I am situated. It would be arrogant of me to suggest that *only* I can see how I am situated. The Department of Health and judges in the UK have been keen to stress that 'best interests' does not mean solely 'best *medical* interests'. I am suggesting that in assessing a person's best interests, the SEA view of the person entails that we should take the broadest possible view of what those interests might be.

I recall a carer of someone with dementia saying to me, in the course of a study on ethical issues for carers (Hughes *et al.* 2002), when we were discussing what might be in the best interests of her husband, 'his best interests are mine and mine are his'. To my mind, this was in no way inappropriate on her part, but rather a realistic comment on the reality of the nature of her and her husband's position as situated individuals whose lives were entwined. But this is not the limit of their situatedness, for it might have been that at some point a doctor, or a social worker, or a judge might have had to insist on something happening to her husband in his best interests that she was *not* happy with. As soon as the notion of 'best interests' is considered in the light of the broader notion of personhood, it is opened up to all of these possibilities. Incidentally, for this reason I think that the way in which the MCA deals with 'best interests' is sensible. Best interests is placed centrally, but is not defined, rather a process for working it out is outlined, but not circumscribed. Well, but what has this to do with end of life?

First, a broad view of best interests commends the holism of the palliative care approach. Perhaps more than any other branch of medicine (although possibly excluding general practice), palliative care has encouraged an holistic approach, where this involves a biological, psychological, social *and spiritual* perspective. The SEA view would add that holism must also take into account cultural, historical, philosophical traditions too, and so on. The palliative care approach, of course, situates the person in the context of family or others. And my experience of palliative care physicians is that they can spend a lot of time clarifying and negotiating what might be best for the person within these often complicated and enmeshed contexts. Good communication is essential because so many end-of-life decisions involve *careful negotiation*, where what is right or wrong has to be *worked out* in a particular context. This is not simply to commend relativism, because the working out and the careful negotiation may be about fixed principles or traditions and how they relate to a particular case.

Second, taking a broad view of best interests, seeing these interests as situated in multifarious ways, involves seeing the person's life historically, as a whole. This means taking seriously their earlier views, as expressed in an advance directive or 'living will' perhaps, but it also means seeing the person's life *now* as relevant and, moreover, it involves seeing his or her life as finite, as a life that will come to an end. Deciding on someone's best interests, therefore, should involve an acceptance of death as a natural part of life. The palliative care approach and the broad view of personhood do not combine to suggest that people should be kept alive at all costs; in fact, just the reverse. But they do combine to suggest that whatever life a person has left should be made as good as possible. In which case, once again, there is no reason why this should not apply to people with dementia too. The argument again comes round to suggesting that, as opposed to the poor standards of care that can often apply, people with dementia should be given a much higher quality of care. At the end of life, they ought to receive good quality specialist palliative dementia care.

In itself a broader view of best interests does not tell us anything about euthanasia or physician-assisted suicide. It might be taken to suggest the possibility that, broadly conceived, a person's best interests might be met by having their 'unbearable suffering' brought to an end by death if no other means were available. Obviously other arguments need to come into play here. I would just observe that if we are talking about allowing the intentional killing of innocent people, our concerns ought to be very broad indeed. One form of arrogance would be to ignore the intolerable suffering of individuals, but another form of arrogance would be to ignore deeply held principles and traditions that have tended to underpin civilized society. Some other accommodation is required and, in my view, the attitudes of palliative care are likely to provide the grounds for alternative solutions.

Intentions and persons

Debates about euthanasia and physician-assisted suicide, especially when discussing the principle of double effect at the end of life, often focus on the notion of intention. According to this principle, it is allowable to do something with foreseen bad consequences if the intention is good. If the aim were good, for instance to relieve the suffering of the dying person, then a foreseen bad consequence, for example the shortening of the person's life, would not be a matter of moral culpability. The distinction between things that are foreseen and things that are intended seems rock solid when we think of much normal medical practice, most prescriptions for instance: the beneficial effects of the prescription are intended, the side effects are not, although they may be foreseen. But the principle of double effect seems laughable if the whole thing hinges on what is going on in a person's head when they act. It sounds as if a doctor might simply make a little speech to him or her self of a particular kind and all will be well, no matter what it is that the doctor is doing. We can even, perhaps, imagine the notorious serial killer Dr Shipman making such little speeches to himself.

Elizabeth Anscombe, the Catholic philosopher friend and executor of Wittgenstein, whose book *Intention* is probably the fullest treatment of the topic, wrote: 'The idea that one can determine one's intentions by making…a little speech to oneself is obvious bosh' (Anscombe 1979, p.42). If the idea of little speeches is to be treated with such derision, what does characterize intention?

The answer is that one has to look towards what is being *aimed at in the action*. It then starts to make sense to speak of the intentional nature of the action, rather than (simply) the intentions of the actor. The two things are not disconnected, but the point is that the actor cannot say that just any old thing was the intention. If at close range I shoot a gun at someone, I am going to have to do a lot of talking to persuade people that this was not a bad action on my part. The action has a certain sort of character, like exploding a bomb on the underground. There may be excuses for shooting someone – it could be the result of a terrible accident of some sort. It is not that the reasons given for doing the action are irrelevant and, similarly, the context is important, but the action itself is of a certain type. The reasons and the type and the context are all going to have to hang together when the action is characterized as an intentional action. Intentions will have to be characterized with a focus on the nature of the action given the particular details of the context. All of this will help to determine the aim of the action, irrespective of any little internal speeches the person might be making.

Elsewhere Anscombe speaks of 'the intention *embodied in* an action' as opposed to 'the further intentions *with* which the action is done' (Anscombe 1981, p.86). The further intentions with which the action is done may be very important, but the notion of the intention embodied in the action leads to the question: 'What intention is inherent in the action you are actually performing?' This is to suggest that an action pursues a particular purpose. So, if

I undertake an action of this particular kind, in some sense it is my intention to pursue this particular purpose (whatever I have said to myself in my head).

To cut to the chase if, thus characterized, an action is intrinsically wrong, I cannot appeal to any little speeches I might have made to myself in order to justify the action. 'I intended to relieve the person's unbearable suffering' or 'I intended to respect the person's previously expressed autonomous wishes' do not look like reasonable arguments if the particular action is of a kind the purpose of which we would normally condemn. The intention *embodied in* the action, that is, might be one that could not normally be tolerated by a moral society.

All of this relates to the SEA view of the person because this view is, in part, supported by the externalist view of the mind, which we have discussed in Chapters 3 and 9, according to which the mind is best characterized by the way it involves the world. So, in understanding persons we move from internal cognitive processes, of remembering or intending, to the world in which the person is embedded. Similarly, intentions cannot be understood as if they were no more than the internal speeches we make to ourselves. They are understood in the world where actions are actions of a certain sort depending in part on the specific purposes they might embody.

What all of this should suggest is that there are grounds for being sceptical when we are told that euthanasia and physician-assisted suicide are all right because of the good intentions of the doctors doing the killing. Instead we should look at the nature of the actions themselves. And doing this might also mean that the person's autonomous wishes must be viewed within a broader context in which human actions are judged according to the intentions they embody. I am taking it that the deliberate, intentional killing of innocent human beings is always wrong. In this I reflect the view of the 1994 House of Lords Select Committee when they said that the prohibition of intentional killing 'is the cornerstone of law and of social relationships' (Lord Walton 1994). Once a particular act of killing is characterized as the deliberate, intentional killing of an innocent person – and I think active voluntary euthanasia and physician-assisted suicide could both be characterized in this way – it would become, in my view, an immoral act of great seriousness.

I shall not try to defend this view further. If I were to do so, I think I would wish to argue that human life itself is a good. I would argue that we should be aiming at enhancing human life, not at its destruction. There are various grounds (e.g. theological grounds) on which the claim that human life is a good might be defended. What I would point to, however, are the instinctive, the natural reactions of carers – family and other non-professional carers as well as professional carers – towards people with even quite severe dementia. They see something worthwhile in their caring role. They see the individual person, however impaired.

It is difficult to be more precise about this. So much of it might be argued away as *merely* reflecting sentimentality or psychological factors, which could in principle be dealt with by appropriate therapy. Some family carers, for instance, find it extremely difficult to take a holiday when the person they care for is in long-term care, even if the person with dementia is not particularly physically ill at the time. Under some circumstances this might, indeed, be pathological. Under other circumstances it reflects tremendous love and nothing more. But I do not wish to get into these details. My point is that these instinctual reactions to care are ubiquitous: amongst families, amongst nurses and other healthcare professionals, amongst different cultures. We see them everyday on our wards and in our care homes. Now, we can call it *just* instinct, but we might also wish to call it virtuous. It certainly reflects the virtues of charity or compassion. And I take it that the virtues help to define us, in some sense, as moral agents. Thus, these virtues which are so ubiquitous amongst carers of all sorts help to define something about the human condition. There is something about life, however damaged, that seems to be regarded as a good, as something worth caring for (or aiming at), even if at some stage it also seems virtuous to 'let go'.

But 'letting go' does not involve suddenly saying that the good worth caring for, the life of the person with dementia, is no longer worth caring for. This is partly the case because of the persistence of personhood into severe dementia. Nor does it mean, however, that the caring has to be the same as it was before. The person's needs change and may finally only amount to the need for comfort, palliative sedation even, without one having to disallow the persistence of the underlying principle that accounts for the moral importance we attach to the notion of personhood. This underlying principle, it seems to me, reflects our proneness to regard human life, in itself, as a good worth living and dying for. The support and care of families and others towards people with dementia would make little sense if it did not reflect the view that there is something intrinsically good about human life itself. To allow that we should aim to destroy this good would be to undermine the grounds for caring. It would leave no principled reason to oppose non-voluntary euthanasia, once the seemingly (but mistakenly) easy step of active voluntary euthanasia had been taken. It would be to undermine the cornerstone of social relationships.

Conclusion

Whilst I cannot develop this theme, what I have argued in this chapter, on the basis of the SEA view of the person is that personhood persists even into severe dementia, that best interests must be understood as broadly as possible, and that intentions are not just 'inner', but are embedded in a context. I have then proposed three further claims in support of the palliative approach in dementia. First, people with dementia cannot be morally disregarded: they deserve the same sort of care as anyone else. Second, a broad view of best interests commends the holism of palliative care. Third, the judgement of an action must include reference to its intentional nature, which is shown both by context as well as by aim. It is particularly (but not solely) the third claim that counts against the type of killing that occurs in active voluntary euthanasia and physician-assisted suicide. For, such acts always involve the deliberate, intentional killing of innocent people, or in the case of physician-assisted suicide the assistance of such deliberate, intentional killing and not to regard this as wrong is to undermine the basis of our human relationships, which are grounded in a mutual recognition that human life itself is precious, a good worth caring for or aiming at. Instead, we should pursue the ideals and principles of palliative care, easing death, allowing it to occur, but equally trying to make a person's life as good as it can be whilst they still live. In dementia care this would require a significant shift in terms of expertise, attitudes and resources, but it is a shift we should feel morally impelled to make.

PART V

Arts

CHAPTER 13

The Art and Practice of Memory and Forgetting

Julian C. Hughes and Ashley McCormick

Introduction

This chapter emerges from our engagement in a Sciart project entitled 'Memory and Forgetting'. Our thoughts were focused on dementia and the ways in which art and science can contribute in a mutually beneficial way to our understanding of dementia. We shall consider the notions of context, concept, content and concern, whilst making reference to the works of Marcel Duchamp, Antony Gormley, Tatsumi Orimoto and to the writings of Roland Barthes. We shall make connections with the neuropathology and neuroimaging of dementia, and pass comment on mild cognitive impairment. Again in this chapter we shall draw upon the works of the philosophers Heidegger, Merleau-Ponty, Parfit and Wittgenstein. Once again, the conclusion we reach is that art, too, encourages a broad view of the person with dementia in which people are seen as inter-relating and as interconnected. Art exerts a tug on the objectivity of science, which should make us more sensitive to the selfhood of people with dementia.

Background thoughts

In 1930 Wittgenstein wrote:

> A work of art forces us – as one might say – to see it in the right perspective but, in the absence of art, the object is just a fragment

of nature like any other; *we* may exalt it through our enthusiasm but that does not give anyone else the right to confront us with it. (I keep thinking of one of those insipid snapshots of a piece of scenery which is of interest for the man who took it because he was there himself and experienced something; but someone else will quite justifiably look at it coldly, in so far as it is ever justifiable to look at something coldly.) (Wittgenstein 1980, pp.4–5)

This gives us the idea of art as a way of seeing (or hearing etc.) that goes beyond the ordinary seeing of everyday life. Science, on the other hand, *might* be regarded as a way of seeing things as ordinary rather than as extraordinary. A scientific explanation, on this view, is a way of simplifying the world. Wittgenstein went on to write: 'Man has to awaken to wonder – and so perhaps do peoples. Science is a way of sending him to sleep again' (p.5)

In the same passage it seems clear that Wittgenstein's complaint is not that science has no possibility of inducing wonder, but that 'the *spirit* in which science is carried on' is not compatible with emotions such as fear or wonder.

One rationale for the sort of Sciart project we were involved in, therefore, in which scientists and artists are brought together to consider a theme from their differing perspectives, is that the artistic understanding of the theme might help to engender, or re-engender, a sense of wonder that may have been lost by the typically reductionist treatment that constitutes a scientific explanation. An alternative rationale, somewhat contrary to Wittgenstein's suggestion, is that science is so full of wonderful discoveries it cannot help but inspire the artist. Our reflections on the Sciart project in which we were engaged during 2002–3 on the themes of 'Memory and Forgetting' are perhaps instructive in that, to an extent, they support both rationales. There was a mutual sharing in terms of our understanding. There was an output in the form of an exhibition, but we also benefited from the extended dialogue that led to our understanding of the themes (Hughes and McCormick 2003). The exhibition was a manifestation of this interaction, which involved give and take from our different perspectives.

For me the most vital thing that art does is recognise the seemingly mundane and everyday as the stuff that is extraordinary and unique, since it is both the source and the result of the stories we tell that allow us to make sense of our lives, stories that allow us to describe ourselves back to ourselves. If art can make a space where lived experience and the imaginary come together to tell us things we don't yet know, then education within art practice is a continual process of give and take, a two-way stretch between the practitioner and other interested parties. (Ainley 2001, pp.89–90)

In the following pages we shall expand on the shared understanding that came from the give and take of our discussions about memory and forgetting.

There are two further background thoughts. First, it is more accurate to describe this as a *clinart* project, because in our case it brought together a clinician and an artist. The difference between the clinical perspective and the scientific perspective is worth pondering briefly. Medical clinicians will inevitably have a scientific understanding of the problems around memory and forgetting. However, they will also have an understanding that is located in the world in which people struggle with memory and forgetting. The biological pull of the basic sciences tends towards the reductionist view: that deficits in terms of recall memory are accounted for by deficits in neurotransmitters, such as acetylcholine, and, for instance, by atrophy of the hippocampus in the medial temporal lobe of the brain. But the clinical reality is that deficits in recall memory cause practical problems in the home and for the family. So there is a natural pull, for the clinician, back towards the context of the community. Similarly, for a public artist, art involves a process of creative relationships with the constituents of different communities (e.g. in Ashley's case this has involved interactions with BMX riders in Cornwall, second-hand car dealers in Essex, traveller and gypsy communities in Cardiff). Socially engaged practice is defined by an ambition to create interventions in both the physical and social fabric of the public realm. Hence, in this project the locus of our normal work, which helps to define our points of view, was already shared, so that our shared understanding was, perhaps, achieved with more facility than might otherwise have been the case.

Second, this shared understanding seems neither to be a matter of science nor of art. It is philosophical. It is at the level of thought. This chapter develops these thoughts. In the passage with which we commenced, Wittgenstein concluded:

> But it seems to me too that there is a way of capturing the world sub specie aeterni other than through the work of the artist. Thought has such a way – so I believe – it is as though it flies above the world and leaves it as it is – observing it from above, in flight. (Wittgenstein 1980, p.5)

This seems a little grandiloquent, but we would agree with the idea that thought is another way of capturing the world. However, these thoughts are not intended to leave the world as it is; they are intended to encourage a broader, more humanistic view of how to consider people with dementia.

Context

The importance of context for a work of art is easily appreciated. There are, at least, two aspects to this: first, the physical space in which art is exhibited or in which it takes place makes a difference to the work of art; second, the context is a cultural and social space created by the artist, but also by those around, for instance the critics or admirers. A particular sculpture will be seen differently in different geographical places, but the artist can also help to create the context that, in turn, creates the aesthetic – more or less successfully. In 1917, Marcel Duchamp created a scandal by sending a porcelain urinal to an exhibition in New York, which he had signed 'R. Mutt'. Clearly these objects, which he claimed could be seen in plumbers' shop windows, could not everywhere be considered as works of art, but the context could make them more than just a piece of plumbing. We should note that the context was not just the hanging of the urinal in the exhibition (in fact it was rejected by the committee), but the story attached to it and the involvement of the artist. The world of art continues to shock or annoy many by its habit of elevating something ordinary to the status of something extraordinary – a habit that amounts to a change of context.

How then does this relate to dementia? During our collaboration, in our discourse, in our arrangements and plans, in our travels, we were *constantly* forgetful or disoriented. We would not accept that this evidence of cognitive dysfunction demonstrated pathology. It is not that our forgetfulness was without significance: it led to wasted time, repetition and embarrassment. Rather, the context meant that our forgetfulness could be excused and laughed off. Forgetting is not in itself pathological and may even be therapeutic or, at least, protective. For forgetfulness to be pathological, it must have a certain history and certain consequences. The occasional forgetfulness of teenagers simply causes parents ire, whereas the occasional forgetfulness of someone in their seventies causes anxiety, if not to the person, then perhaps to the children. And a pattern of forgetfulness, with the emergence of other impairments, is a cause for concern, at some point.

The 'at some point' suggests the importance of context. If the context were the neuropathology laboratory, the 'at some point' in relation to the forgetfulness of Alzheimer's dementia would refer *inter alia* to a specific number of senile plaques (one of the hallmarks of Alzheimer's dementia) found in the cerebral cortex. The number of such plaques required has, of course, been correlated with the severity of dementia. Hence we can say, pointing down the microscope, that at *this* point the diagnosis of definite Alzheimer's disease has been made. The problem is, however, there will be marginal cases and the real context must be the clinical one. As we know from the famous 'Nun study', pathology does not correlate in an exact manner with symptoms: some of the nuns in this study had pathology but no significant symptoms or signs and others had obvious cognitive impairment but minimal pathology (Snowdon 2003). What counts in the end, despite the hard concreteness of neuropathology, is what the person actually does in the world (Hughes *et al.* 2006).

Recognizing the importance of context does not suggest that there is no such thing as dementia, but it does show how any particular episode of forgetfulness, as it were outside the flow of life, might be irrelevant. This suggests some important insights of a clinical nature that can be derived from our ponderings on art. We suggested in relation to art that there were two aspects (at least) to context. The first was the physical context or space, the gallery in which Duchamp wished to place his urinal. The second was the social context created by the artist and others; for instance, the socio-cultural reaction to Duchamp's urinal. It is for this second reason that trying to pass off a urinal *now* as a work of art would seem lame: it would just be imitation.

Forgetfulness and context also have these two features. There is the space in which the person is forgetful. This may be very important, but (at least in theory) the space can be made safe. If a person were only forgetful in safe places, the consequences would be less serious. The real issue of significance for us, however, is the social or cultural context of forgetfulness. This context is seen from without and from within and there may or may not be congruence between these views: others may be very concerned and the person less so, or vice versa, or the concern might be equally shared, or it might be absent. But the question about when forgetfulness is pathological arises again. At some point a line can be drawn, but now the 'at some point' is not a number of senile plaques: instead the line is drawn according to the degree of concern. Pathological forgetfulness seems to be akin to a social construct.

Even if we step back from the suggestion that dementia is socially constructed (Thornton 2006), we are left with the insight from thinking about art, namely that forgetfulness – whether or not it is pathological – has to be judged in a social context. And whether or not the person's forgetfulness is a problem must be decided in the course of everyday life. *This* will not simply be a matter of counting senile plaques. Now there is a way in which the point about context is mundane: everything is, of course, understood in a social context. The point here, however, is that, in the case of dementia, the context is often problematic: it is the socio-cultural response that leads to at least some of the disability (or handicap) associated with dementia. For example, the new 'diagnosis' of mild cognitive impairment (MCI) pathologizes forgetfulness, by placing it in a medical context. This may be problematic, not just conceptually, but for the people concerned and for our whole way of thinking about ageing (Bavidge 2006).

MCI is regarded as a potential pre-dementia state (O'Brien and Grayson 2013). It is characterized by a subjective complaint of forgetfulness without other (more global) impairments. The problem is that, whilst each year a proportion of people with MCI convert to dementia (by developing cognitive problems in other domains, such as deficits in orientation, or language, or praxis), a proportion do not. So some people with MCI remain merely forgetful. The worry here is three-fold. First, to give a 'diagnosis' that may appear to condemn the person to the intolerable life of dementia seems unethical if it is not actually so. Second, even if the person *is* going to develop dementia, it may be that stigmatizing him or her early on by applying this label is unhelpful, even if it allows the person to arrange his or her affairs. But, third, the whole endeavour – the whole research industry around MCI (the search for genetic markers or for brain dysfunction on neuroimaging etc.) – misses the point of context.

The point is that the real issue is one to do with values. Do we need to know what comes before dementia (the pharmaceutical industry might think that we do, but given the current lack of a cure this seems debatable)? Do we want to see minimal forgetfulness in old age as a condition or disease, rather than as simply a way of life that can be 'laughed off' as we 'laugh off' forgetfulness at a younger age? Do we wish this sort of forgetfulness to be viewed as a medical problem, rather than as a social phenomenon to be handled in mundane ways by social support and reassurance? It may be that all these things should be so, but it is important to see that the questions are raised within a context of values where there may well be some disagreement.

The search for MCI is part and parcel of what Sabat (2001) calls 'defectology'. Neuropsychologists can find defects by their cognitive tests and these then help to define the condition. In so doing, however, the tests are in danger of missing the person in the human context. In our project, for instance, a key partner was Mr B, who was a self-taught amateur photographer. He had been taking pictures for more than 45 years and had an archive of many thousands of slides. At the time of the exhibition he had mild to moderate Alzheimer's disease (way beyond MCI), yet in conversations he was animated and informative. His language problems meant that he stumbled over words and would drift through a range of subjects. He had used his slides over many years to give shows to audiences in social clubs and residential homes. He regarded these shows as journeys. His slides were used in the 'Memory and Forgetting' exhibition, with his collaboration, to evoke themes, forms, colours and visual puns in ways that suggested order and disorder. In the course of this collaboration Mr B's individuality and enthusiasm predominated, because of the social context, despite his brain pathology. Meanwhile, his slides took on a greater significance and aesthetic because of their associations with Mr B. The slide show had some sort of personal significance too for the audience who undertook a journey from their own perspective whilst watching the matched pairs of his slides appear, disappear and gradually come round again.

Concept

Modern art is sometimes clearly conceptual, but even when it is representational it usually carries a concept, either overtly or covertly. In thinking about 'Memory and Forgetting' we discussed the phenomenon of art as commemoration. Memorials are by far the most common form of public art; so much so that as a group they tend to blur with the urban background. They become invisible and, paradoxically, forgotten. Even so, the preoccupation with such objects continues, as debates around memorials to Princess Diana in London and to 9/11 at Ground Zero demonstrate. There have been several monuments erected in Newcastle to individuals, typically male, who have contributed to society. Particular attributes have been deemed suitable for commemoration, such as those of the hero (valour, courage and sacrifice) or those of the benefactor (kindness, wealth and generosity).

A rough and ready consultation exercise on the streets of Newcastle showed that out of about 20 individuals, 75 per cent did not know anything about the subjects represented by the memorials they were passing. In the main, then, the memorials were anonymous, or what they commemorated was forgotten. We originally toyed with the concept of comparing public memorials with the sort of private mementos that fill the rooms of residents of homes for people with dementia. But we also viewed different forms of brain scan, in particular SPECT (single photon emission computed tomography) scans. To the clinical scientist's eye these convey a picture of brain function or dysfunction, but to an artist they were also a representation of something forgotten: a forgotten thought perhaps in the scanner. As seen on the computer screen, they were also anonymous representations of a person's now inaccessible mental life. The idea of capturing this on photographic paper and the idea of forgotten mementos led to the concept of capturing forgotten objects by such a form of representation.

Memory function itself is sometimes thought of in terms of storage and retrieval processes. Wards looking after people with dementia, in a similar way, have systems for the storage and retrieval of lost property. But the property is seldom retrieved. In the lost property of a particular ward, amongst many things, lost glasses predominated. These were placed into a tangle (to be redolent of the neurofibrillary tangles seen in the brains of patients with Alzheimer's) and, without any form of camera (in contrast to the gamma camera used to create SPECT scans), a photogram was constructed and entitled 'no ifs, ands, or buts', which is itself a parody of an element from a well-known assessment of cognitive function. Hundreds of these photograms were then reproduced and handed out as mementos of the exhibition. So the simple representation of the forgotten glasses hides a complex story of thoughts and ideas. But, inevitably, the full thought behind the concept, even if some of it were overt, was hidden and will, in turn, be forgotten.

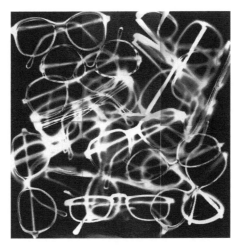

Figure 13.1 'no ifs, ands, or buts'
by Ashley McCormick

There are two interesting thoughts to consider. Roland Barthes, in *Camera Lucida* wrote: 'in Photography I can never deny that *the thing has been there*. There is a superimposition here: of reality and of the past' (Barthes 2000, p.76). The first thought, therefore, concerns the idea of photographic representation. The second thought, linked to the first, concerns the degree to which the brain scans and the photograms operate as portraits, illuminating something forgotten of the history and personality of an anonymous subject.

The photogram is a reality, but it also represents the past. Barthes says that a photograph is never in essence a memory. In fact, he says, a photograph blocks memory: it 'fills the sight by force' (2000, p.91). But it is always about what has been there, even if it has passed, or is dead. The photograph is, after all, a highly scientific or technological thing to do with chemicals and light; whilst at the same time it is a way of trying to capture something subjective. Barthes describes himself having a debate about science and subjectivity and arriving at what he calls a 'curious notion', namely: 'Why mightn't there be, somehow, a new science for each object?' (Barthes 2000, p.8). He spent some while looking for a photograph of his mother that would not just provoke her identity, but also what he called her truth. After numerous mundane photographs he found one which 'was indeed essential, it achieved for me, utopically, *the impossible science of the unique being*' (p.71). The photogram of the tangled, forgotten glasses does not convey a unique being, nor do the SPECT scans but, akin to Barthes's conclusion about photography, they do show that a person has been there '*in flesh and blood*' (p.79).

To return to dementia, the photogram is a memorial (not a memory) of real people and real lives. These were lives that interconnected with other lives. Choices were made, about glasses, and there was a story that led to the ward and the loss of the glasses. Our reflections have been conceptual. They have revealed, through a discussion of photographic representation and the place of memorials, something of the thing represented. The essence of photography, 'that-has-been', leads back to a notion of real people, '*in flesh and blood*', interconnecting and pursuing their lives beyond the picture, in a world of others.

The simple parallel being drawn between dementia and art is that they both involve conceptual thought. The ways in which art is conceptual are readily apparent, even if the concepts are sometimes opaque. Reflection on the conceptual character of art achieves two things. First, the concepts in art characteristically say something about the human condition, or at least the world as experienced by human beings. The examples we have considered point towards the ways in which we are characteristically positioned as beings that interact with the world and with others. This is no less the case for people with dementia. Our interactions, however, should be positive and enhancing where the person's condition increases his or her vulnerability. Memory and forgetting link us to other people (conceptually and in reality), but these links may be fragile, so they may need to be handled carefully, with concern or what Heidegger (1962) called solicitude. Second, reflection on the conceptual character of art leads us to a recognition of how the notions of memory and forgetting are themselves conceptual and, as such, tied to a surround (a context) in order for them to have meaning (or content). In this way, the pull of conceptual understanding is in the direction of social context, culture and history, and away from a disconnected, atomistic and (narrowly) 'scientific' view of the phenomena. In short, the influence of art tugs us from the technological to the narrative of real individuals.

Content

As we have seen in earlier chapters, it is sometimes argued in connection with dementia that the person no longer exists because he or she cannot remember. But this account of both personhood and dementia is contradicted by accounts that regard personhood as involving more than just memory. Instead, the alternative account stresses the extent to which the person cannot be circumscribed, because of his or her situatedness in an individual, but multi-layered, context involving personal, historical, cultural, social, psychological, moral and spiritual fields, etcetera. The SEA view of the person revives the idea that, even in severe dementia, it still makes sense to talk of the person, because of the various ways in which personhood can survive through the body and within a context of caring others.

As we have also seen, the externalist account of the mind also suggests that memories are essentially shareable or public (whether or not they actually are shared or public). Again, this locates the person with memories within an embedding context. This whole way of thinking, as we saw in Chapter 3, breaks down the distinction between inner things and outer things. It is not that we have to deny that there are inner processes altogether, it is just that we should not make the mistake of thinking that remembering is solely an inner process (Wittgenstein 1968, §§305–6). Not only are memories in principle shareable, but also – as it happens – that we have remembered certain things *can* be seen outwardly. Think, for instance, of the man with marked dementia with no language and dependent on others for all of his personal needs, whose face lights up when his wife visits the home where he lives.

The broader view of the person, which relies on a breaking down of the distinction between the inner and the outer, is supported by the work of the sculptor Antony Gormley. He stresses the importance of the body (and the skin) as the site of interaction with the world. Through the outer body he conveys inner subjectivity:

> Gormley, like Merleau-Ponty, is much drawn to the idea of correspondence between the visible and invisible; he has also said that his interest in the body was aroused because embodiment, or being-in-the-world, provided him with a way of escaping from the dualism of dialectics. In other words, to Gormley the body is the articulation of meaning; it is that in which sense is given and out of which sense emerges. (Hutchinson 2000, p.42)

The body as the articulation of meaning suggests that in dementia, even where effective language has been lost, there is still a point to attending to gestures and sound. Moreover, there are other reasons for thinking that the loss of cognitive processes does not affect the potential for emotional expression and conative drives. It may be that the *intensity* of the person's subjective experience can still be conveyed and should be taken seriously, because, amongst other reasons, the person with dementia, as a situated embodied agent, is still a being-in-the-world.

As Gormley says:

> I am interested in something that one could call the collective subjective. I really like the idea that if something is intensely felt by one individual that intensity can be felt even if the precise cause of the intensity is not recognised. I think that is to do with the equation that I am trying to make between an individual, highly personal experience and this very objective thing – a thing in the world, amongst other things. (Gombrich and Gormley 2000, pp.18–19)

The person, as a body, is in the world and it is this spatio-temporal reality that conveys the shareable inner life. Gormley's talk of the 'collective subjective' is akin to the idea of human consciousness developed in Chapter 9: it is not the self-consciousness of the individual. Rather, it reflects the shared nature of our 'inner' lives. But that inner reality, as Wittgenstein suggests, 'has meaning only in the stream of life' (Wittgenstein 1992, p.30). There is a sense in which those around must also maintain meaning.

Concern

In the 'Memory and Forgetting' exhibition there was a small piece in which an illuminated line was modified by the voice of Joan, a lady with severe dementia who could not speak. Yet she could sing. Her family and carers had evolved a way of receiving that was respectful and open-hearted, which encouraged her to sing with them songs such as 'It's a long way to Tipperary'. This was a meaningful activity for Joan and is an example of carers indulging in meaning-making (Widdershoven and Berghmans 2006) in a way that facilitated pleasurable emotional exchange despite Joan's cognitive disabilities.

For Heidegger,

> 'concern' is understood in a very general sense as covering the almost endless ways in which man's interests impinge on the beings around him... To be in the world is to be concerned with the world, to be engaged in ceaseless interaction with the things we find within the world. (Macquarrie 1972, p.84)

But, as distinct from the 'concern' by which we relate to things in the world, personal concern or 'solicitude' characterizes relations between selves. 'An authentic solicitude for the other helps him to his freedom and to his own unique possibilities for selfhood' (Macquarrie 1968, p.18).

Joan's sisters and carers were open to her as a person and she clearly flourished in response to their solicitude or care. But the possibility that she could instead have been regarded as not worth interacting with, as not worth being given scope for her free expression, which she clearly enjoyed, is real in the field of dementia care.

In the art of Tatsumi Orimoto the notion of engagement with the world is apparent in his live art events in public settings where he appears with a mask made of bread, often escorted by other *Breadmen*. These performances, in public settings, involve the artist's own body as part of the performance and involve an interaction with those around him. Tatsumi Orimoto has also produced a series of photographs, called *Art Mama*, of his mother who has Alzheimer's disease. He has recorded her everyday routines in which she becomes a living sculpture. He demonstrates by these photographs his close relationship with his mother (as shown in Figure 13.2), but he also comments on the treatment of older people in an increasingly individualistic society, which is less open to the interconnectivity and mutuality implied by the Heideggerian analysis of the human existent as essentially 'concerned'.

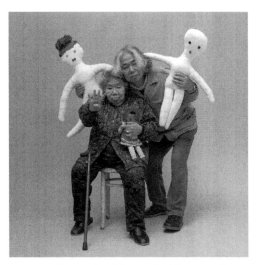

Figure 13.2 From *Art Mama*, by Tatsumi Orimoto

Tatsumi also uses his art, which he takes to institutions for people with dementia, to stimulate and inspire the residents. He describes how, with his type of provocative exchange – for example he puts huge shoes on their feet – he can make the people with Alzheimer's regain some vitality through interaction.

Similarly, the ways in which activities involving art, or indeed any meaningful activities, can sustain and re-invigorate the selfhood of others is powerfully captured in the photography of Cathy Greenblat (2012). So, too, in the communicative techniques of John Killick and Kate Allan (Killick and Allan 2001) and the recognition that creativity and communication go hand in hand

(Killick and Craig 2012), in the possibilities for creative activity stressed by John Zeisel in his work involving museums (Zeisel 2009), in the possibilities revealed by dance (Coaten 2002) or by music (Clair and Memmott 2008) and by the creative arts in general (Hayes and Povey 2011), we see the possibility of enhancing the well-being and standing of people with dementia.

Once again, it is by interaction and concern – which we have seen is typical of public art performances, and for which a philosophical account can be given in terms of our mutual dependency as human existents in the world – that people with dementia can be seen as individuals with the potential still to be engaged within the human world.

Summary

So, one conclusion from the 'Memory and Forgetting' project is that artists and clinicians (and scientists) can usefully talk to each other in a way that is beneficial. In so doing, in relation to what it is to remember or to forget, they broaden the view. Forgetting is seen as located in a context of values. Contentful memory is seen as itself a shareable feature of the world. People are regarded, at a conceptual level, as interconnected subjectively by their objective, bodily presence. And people with dementia should evoke our concern in a way that reflects our mutual standing with them, and sensitivity to them, as situated embodied agents, rather than as objects solely for pity or even disrespect (Post 2006).

Ashley McCormick – biographical details

Ashley McCormick is an artist, curator and educator. She is committed to developing inspiring collaborative creative projects and events, which value and broaden the interests, imaginations, skills and experiences of diverse partners and audiences.

Graduating from the Royal College of Art in 1995, Ashley became an Associate Partner with muf architecture/art from 1996 to 2005. Since then she has worked as collaborator, consultant and facilitator with a number of other artists, architecture practices,

organizations and institutions including the London Legacy Development Corporation, erect architecture, East architecture/landscape/urban design, Gort Scott architects, Tate Britain, Camden Art Centre, Design for London, Bow Arts Trust, The Building Exploratory, Surestart, Creative Partnerships and English Heritage.
www.ashleymccormickprojects.co.uk

CHAPTER 14

In Praise of 'Negative Capability'

Keats and Killick

The poet John Keats (1795–1821) wrote to his brothers in December 1817 to praise the idea of 'negative capability'. He described this as 'when man is capable of being in uncertainties, Mysteries, doubts, without any irritable reaching after fact & reason…' (Keats 1990, p.370). In this brief chapter I shall argue – or rather I wish to sketch a picture, without irritably reaching for facts or reasons – that our approach to dementia is (or should be) above all an aesthetic one. It is (or should be) about how we see the world, and my contention is that we should see the world in terms of beauty, so our approach to dementia could be a matter of searching for beauty; it could be a matter of good taste, of searching for joy even.

This might induce outrage, for how could dementia be a matter of joy? Even if it can sometimes be relatively benign, it is more usually a source of sadness because of the inherent sense of loss and distress that accompanies dementia and, in its severer forms, it is a cruel and painful condition. But I did not say that *dementia* was a matter of joy, rather *our approach* to dementia should be a matter of *looking* for joy. This followed my contention that we should see the world in terms of beauty and is based on a recognition that dementia is in-the-world. I am reaching after neither fact nor reason, but an aesthetic perception of the world, which reacts to beauty as (according to Keats in the opening lines of *Endymion*) 'a joy forever'.

The notion of an *approach to dementia* is, of course, rather an impersonal thing; we are really interested in our approach to *real people with dementia*. Then several things become easier to accept all at once. In our relationships with people we must often be struck by something that is essentially unknowable about them. Albeit they are just like us, we never really know what it is like to be The Other. Here are 'uncertainties, Mysteries, doubts'. Yet there is, at the same time, something that *is* known. The more we know her – the more we can look into her eyes and hold our mutual gaze – the more there is something communicated and shared. We might be inclined to say that whatever it is, it is meaningful. It conveys some form of truth, which in turn can be conceived as something beautiful. Thus, we are at the heart of 'negative capability':

> 'Beauty is truth, truth beauty', – that is all
> Ye know on earth, and all ye need to know.

> (Keats 1990, p.289)

Our approach to the world, which includes our approach to real people even with dementia who are in-the-world, is not (I want to say) fundamentally scientific, factual, reasoned; no, it is more a matter of intuition, of sharing knowledge that cannot be spoken, of appreciation. It is a matter of grasping unuttered truths and of seeing something which is ultimately mysterious and cannot be pinned down. Our reaction to the world is fundamentally aesthetic, even when – in scientific mode – we are 'reaching after fact & reason'. If Keats started his adult life as a physician, who had to learn the facts of anatomy and the reasons behind pathophysiology, his mature inclination was to grasp the world in a manner that was altogether more sensual:

> O, let me once more rest
> My soul upon that dazzling breast!
> Let once again these aching arms be plac'd,
> The tender gaolers of thy waist!
> And let me feel that warm breath here and there
> To spread a rapture in my very hair, –
> O, the sweetness of the pain,

Give me those lips again!
Enough! Enough! it is enough for me
To dream of thee!

(Keats 1990, p.329)

This is not the world of hypercognitivism (Post 1995), but the world of embodied selfhood (Kontos 2004), where the person is broadly conceived as a situated embodied agent (Hughes 2001b). This is where we grasp our experience of the world as sensual as much as it is rational. As Keats famously exclaimed to his friend Benjamin Bailey in a letter in 1817: 'O for a Life of Sensations rather than of Thoughts' (1990, p.365).

John Killick might have used this as his motto for his work with people with dementia, in which he has engaged with them through various art forms and more recently through play (Killick 2013a). In the Introduction to his recent book, *Dementia Positive*, he has written: 'We are dealing with, on the one hand, possibly the most complex condition humans can face, and on the other, individuals in all their diversity. So this is a book of hints and potentials, not certainties' (Killick 2013b, p.13). Killick thus embraces the possibilities of negative capability.

The idea I wish to acknowledge as key is that, even in the presence of cognitive impairment, the person with dementia remains an aesthetic being where the possibility of interaction persists through words and poetry, through painting or pottery, or any other form of human creativity. Killick stands, therefore, shoulder to shoulder with the likes of Tom Kitwood (1997), who emphasized the PERSON with dementia, with Stephen Post (2006), who highlights the emotional and relational nature of human beings, with Steve Sabat (2001), who has demonstrated so well the importance of engagement with the person with dementia in a way that is reaffirming, and so on. This is the new culture of dementia care. It is a psychosocial approach, where this does not mean that the biological facts are irrelevant, but where they are not regarded as the whole deal. They sit in a context, which I am characterizing as essentially aesthetic. My dementia means that there are things I cannot do, but there are still things that I *can* do and there are still things that are important to me. Looking for the possibility of human flourishing, which is often to be found in relationships, could be regarded as an aesthetic endeavour. Understanding a person's meaning through creative practices can be thought of as a matter of looking for beauty.

Glimpses

to see what is beautiful
to hear what is beautiful
they don't know what is beautiful

all these young people
good men, nice boys, fine chaps –
they are too busy to see

it'll be a good bit longer
before you see
what you want to see

but they don't want to see
what in some queer way
they are anxious to see

we see it very rarely
but the difference is
we are trying to see!

(from Killick and Cordonnier 2000)

Knowing another person, making a connection, being in the moment with them, these possibilities are joyful. But there is also something mysterious. It is the mystery that surrounds the effects of art, of music say, and its ability to convey meaning. How does a look convey meaning so powerfully? How does a musical phrase or a poem? Getting to know someone with dementia involves the same (or similar) intuitions, reactions and sensibilities. And contact with an Other at this sort of level can also be described as a spiritual experience. It contains the 'Mystery' that Keats intended by the notion of 'negative capability'. So our engagements are not just psychosocial affairs; the required approach to the person with dementia is also spiritual. Killick describes the deep level of communication that can be achieved through being 'in the moment' with another and then says of such an instance of intimacy that it reflects 'a profound interconnectedness with another human being, which enriched our lives and, though we cannot prove this, the lives of those with whom we interacted' (Killick 2011, p.60). He went on to say:

> From observation of people with dementia in hospitals, nursing homes and in their own homes, I would suggest that most people with the condition are currently being denied the opportunity to interact in spiritual ways. Their lives seem to be confined to the mundane... What is needed is supporters...prepared to take the risk involved in deep communication and surrender to the moment. (p.60)

Speaking of a similar encounter, with an Australian woman who had advanced dementia and had not spoken for some years, who none the less engaged in an albeit inarticulate conversation with John, he and Kate Allan have elsewhere written of:

> a capacity which acquires ever greater importance in interactions with persons with dementia, that of being *in the moment* with our attention fully and open-mindedly focused on the person and our encounter with them. (Allan and Killick 2010, pp.223–4)

Thus, 'uncertainties, Mysteries, doubts, without any irritable reaching after fact & reason' lie close to the heart of our abilities to communicate as human beings generally; but particularly close to the heart of the possibility of communication with people with dementia. And in searching for this we are searching for the possibility of joy and beauty: this is an aesthetic endeavour.

It is also one that privileges relationships and our interconnectedness, which can be achieved through artistic creativity. In the Sciart project described in the previous chapter (see also Hughes and McCormick 2003), we were intrigued by the way so many things are routinely forgotten: we ourselves were constantly forgetting meetings and the like, seemingly without 'uncertainties' or 'doubts'. Ashley drew attention to the ways in which public memorials often seem to disappear, to become taken for granted in our public spaces. What they commemorate is often forgotten. As part of the project Ashley arranged one evening for the plinth of the Earl Grey Monument at the heart of Newcastle to be illuminated with text that was kindly supplied by John Killick, from the poem *Nae Oniebody*:

I'm no' a man, neither resident nor staff.
I'm no' ma god-daughter, and she's no' me either.

. . .

I'm no' needin' a glass o' orange for a laxative 'cos I'm corkit.
I'm no' the tail o' ma nightie that's wringin' wet, nor ma bottom sheet.

. . .

I'm no' ma feet, nor ma features, nor' what grows on 'em.
I'm no a bottom more nor onie man in this whoreshole.

This that I've told you is all that I can give.
But I have a name – I'm 'Jack in the Beanstalk'.
It belongs to me, but I'm nae oniebody in it.

(from Killick and Cordonnier 2000)

But on the night of this event in Newcastle another took place, which was a protest against the war in Iraq, which was about to commence. The demonstrators congregated around the Earl Grey Monument and the words of a Scottish woman with dementia (who wrote down *Nae Oniebody* with John), shone through the crowd and onto the monument, on which graffiti was also being inscribed. Some thought the words were to do with the protest or were a form of some other protest. Some read the words with attention. Others ignored them, but were bemused. Others did not notice that there was anything else happening at all. There was, then, a sense of confusion, but also a sense that things fitted together in an inchoate manner.

We are interconnected. When something bad happens anywhere, it affects us all. The aesthetic sense is also one that makes us want to cry out because of a lack of beauty. Where is justice? Where are joy and love? Whatever the rights and wrongs of war in general, or of that war in particular, the doubts and uncertainties that characterize negative capability are also to be found in our reactions to anything that involves harm to others. Even if we feel we must act definitively on occasions, to invade a country's air space or to deprive a person of their liberty (by putting them in a nursing home against their wishes say), our approach must reflect our background standing as interdependent human beings in the world, whose inherent propensity to flourish through artistic creativity should make us open to the requirement that we seek joy and not its opposite, beauty and not its opposite; we should seek hope, truth, love, peace and so on. The aesthetic approach should mean that we pursue even our certainties with uncertainty, with an openness to better possibilities.

Elsewhere, having described the work of John and Kate, I have argued that we need not just a new culture of dementia care, but a revolution: 'The revolution required at the personal level is to make our human encounters matter in an authentic way' (Hughes 2011a, p.244). Creativity can encourage authentic communication. Having a sense of the mystery of human interactions should encourage us to look at others more intensely, with a keener eye for the sparks that unite us humanly. So, too, we should listen more carefully to what is being said, to the poetry that inhabits our ways of making meaning, however impaired they might be. This is not easy in our current cultures of care, where the emphasis is on efficiency and effective protocols. This is far removed from being-with-the-Other-in-the-moment in an authentic way. Hence, we need a revolution. But perhaps it is more realistic to consider that the revolution might come in small steps.

The work of John Killick has shown us how our approach to people with dementia can be and needs to be aesthetic. It has shown us, in a revolutionary manner, that there is another way. We can progress by intuition, despite uncertainties. We can progress by leaving behind our rationality and by taking risks in our meetings with others. The revolution will come if we seek what is true in our encounters and see that this is also something beautiful: 'that is all Ye know on earth, and all ye need to know'.

Conclusion

Care – Solicitude and solidarity

Ageing is often presented as problematic. But a broad view of ageing, which allows it to be seen simply as a manifestation of the lives that we live, should help us to regard old age in a more promising light. There may be problems, but there can be possibilities too, which depend on our attitudes as much as on our bodies. The broad view also embeds our lives in the context of others, so that our social environment will play a considerable role in our ability to age well or poorly. All of this stems from our human nature, not just as biophysical beings, not just as psychologically continuous and connected beings, but as situated embodied agents with the potential to act in and on the world.

As we have seen, a defining feature of our lives is that we are minded, but – more than this – that our minds reach out into the world and interact with others. Indeed, this possibility is constitutive of our being. We are deeply, at a metaphysical level, embedded in the world. This is not simply a physical fact, although it is importantly that too, but a conceptual reality. Our lives are shaped by the world, by our engagements and interactions, and our lives shape the world. Our concern for the world, therefore, is constitutive: it is part of our make-up. This concern stems from our mindedness, from the nature of our thoughts and the ways in which our thoughts and intentions interact with the world. They do this partly through language, which is itself a unique feature of our mindedness and of how that inner world of subjectivity is also outer and always, potentially, shareable, whether in straightforward conversation or through art and music and great literature, but always as a constitutive feature of our being as we are.

Our inner worlds, that is, reach out to the external world. So the worlds of health and social care, as well as the worlds of law and politics, reflect our embodied subjectivities. We are always situated in these broader domains, interconnected with the broader world of others. We cannot avoid this feature of our lives, namely that we exist with others: our being-in-the-world is characterized by this mutual dependency.

Care

In which case, care is not just something that we do internally. It is constitutive that we are in the world with others and the nature of our shared lives means that we are not simply interested in others as sources of amusement, as means to pass the time of day; we are interested in others because of the significance the others inevitably hold for us as beings of this type in the world, as ends in themselves. That significance has a moral or ethical, as well as a political, quality. It is the bedrock of ordinary care. It is not something we can just ignore. To be oblivious to the needs and concerns of others requires a great effort of will, unless we are deficient in some way as a result of illness or viciousness. Solicitude, both as an existential reality and as a way of being, is our more natural reaction to others. It is an existential reality in that our being is, as Heidegger suggests, typically being-with-others. It is a way of being in that, psychologically and socially, we cannot seem to ignore the plight, or even just the lives, of others. Indeed, this awareness may be hard-wired.

Our type of being-in-the-world, therefore, as minded persons, has a number of consequences. First, we cannot show care except by our actions. Care and solicitude are states of mind too, but they are instantiated through our embodied actions. In the absence of actions, care will seem lacking. Second, although our solicitude can be given a metaphysical interpretation, so that it is an intellectual way of appreciating our human nature, it can also be sensual. We have an aesthetic sense of our place in the world with others; and through art, or other manifestations of human beauty, the nature of our solicitude is apprehended as something shared. Third, care is a political matter: it emanates from our standing in the *polis* as persons amongst persons, but it is also a feature of political life itself that it should strive for the common good. There is a right to care and a duty, but these come from our way of being, which includes many other aspects of our lives: our needs, our values, our hopes and our anxieties. They are non-negotiable features of our lives. Solicitude, therefore, is a prerequisite of solidarity, but solidarity is predicated on our solicitude.

If solicitude can be seen as an existential manifestation of *angst*, it can also be seen as a symptom of hope. Our being-in-the-world is eased by the solicitude of others, and by our own solicitude we make the world a better place. Solidarity, meanwhile, helps to build up the stock of good nature in the world through its practical demand for solicitous and careful action. And solidarity and solicitude together require that we pay each other closer attention in our *being-with*. Taking more notice, empathic understanding, seeking out, representing others – these are ways in which we show both our solicitude and solidarity.

How we think about dementia, then, is a matter of real concern. For if we can see it in the broad context of the multidimensional world, in which as minded people our lives must be understood as mutually involving, but also as biopsychosocial and spiritual realities, we are likely both to take the right attitudes towards doing something about dementia from every possible perspective – because we are situated in every possible perspective – but we are also likely to see people with dementia in a better light. There are things that we can do for them, but there are also ways in which the lives of people with dementia are simply lives like any other. They will respond to joy and to laughter, to kindness and to compassion. Our solicitude and solidarity should mean that we wish to do things *now*, which will involve both a call to individual action as well as a call to political action. If people with dementia find it difficult to respond to the world in any way that seems enthusiastic or hopeful, it may be this is because we do not take the risks we should in order to engage with them in a manner that is facilitating. This is a matter of commitment. We know what can be achieved occasionally, but only political and individual commitment will produce the right sort of responses on a larger scale. This will require, however, both a broad view of the problem and a broad view of the potential solutions.

Our care and solicitude must be real. But it cannot be narrowly defined. Nothing is ruled out and everything is ruled in. How we think about dementia just epitomizes how we think about our lives as a whole. Given a sense of wonder at the nature of our being and what this entails, the significance of our lives cannot be underestimated. It may be that we should take a more positive view of dementia. It is, after all, just another way of living, even if it places demands on all those involved. But those demands should be met by a more broadly based solicitude that calls on the whole of society for support, which is the demand for solidarity. How we think about dementia should lead us to view caring for people with dementia as a community endeavour. But we should also recognize the potential that will persist for engagement if we can *be-with* in the right sort of way. We should recognize that our situated nature means that nothing is ever lost completely. Things persist in the memories of those around us and our nexus of narratives, like life itself, persists even if there are losses. Ageing and dementia might bring decay of one sort or another; and yet, to quote William Wordsworth:

> …the wiser mind
> Mourns less for what age takes away
> Than what it leaves behind

> (from *The Fountain*, Wordsworth 2000, p.139)

References

Agich, G.J. (2003) *Dependence and Autonomy in Old Age: An Ethical Framework for Long-Term Care*. Cambridge: Cambridge University Press.

Ainley, R. (ed.) (2001) *This Is What We Do: a muf manual*. London: Ellipsis.

Allan, K. and Killick, J. (2010) 'Communicating with People with Dementia.' In J.C. Hughes, M. Lloyd-Williams and G.A. Sachs (eds) *Supportive Care for the Person with Dementia*. Oxford: Oxford University Press.

American Psychiatric Association (2013) 'Mild Neurocognitive Disorder.' *Diagnostic and Statistical Manual of Mental Disorders (DSM-5)*. Available at www.dsm5.org/Documents/Mild%20Neurocognitive%20Disorder%20Fact%20Sheet.pdf, accessed 6 February 2014.

Anscombe, G.E.M. (1979) *Intention*. Oxford: Blackwell.

Anscombe, G.E.M. (1981) *The Collected Philosophical Papers of G.E.M. Anscombe. Volume Three: Ethics, Religion and Politics*. Oxford: Blackwell.

Aquilina, C. and Hughes, J.C. (2006) 'The Return of the Living Dead: Agency Lost and Found?' In J.C. Hughes, S.J. Louw and S.R. Sabat (eds) *Dementia: Mind, Meaning, and the Person*. Oxford: Oxford University Press.

Baldwin, C. and Capstick, A. (2007) *Tom Kitwood on Dementia: A Reader and Critical Commentary*. Maidenhead: McGraw Hill and Open University Press.

Baldwin, C. and Estey-Burtt, B. (2013) 'The Ethics of Caring.' In T. Dening and A. Thomas (eds) *Oxford Textbook of Old Age Psychiatry*. Oxford: Oxford University Press.

Barthes, R. (2000) *Camera Lucida* (trans. R. Howard). London: Vintage.

Bavidge, M. (2006) 'Ageing and Human Nature.' In J.C. Hughes, S.J. Louw and S.R. Sabat (eds) *Dementia: Mind, Meaning, and the Person*. Oxford: Oxford University Press.

Bellhouse, J., Holland, A. J., Clare, I.C.H., Gunn, M. and Watson, P. (2003a) 'Capacity-based mental health legislation and its impact on clinical practice: 1) Admission to hospital.' *Journal of Mental Health Law 9*, 1, 9–23.

Bellhouse, J., Holland, A.J., Clare, I.C.H., Gunn, M. and Watson, P. (2003b) 'Capacity-based mental health legislation and its impact on clinical practice: 2) Treatment in hospital.' *Journal of Mental Health Law 9*, 1, 24–37.

Berlinger, N., Jennings, B. and Wolf, S.M. (2013) *The Hastings Center Guidelines for Decisions on Life-Sustaining Treatment and Care Near the End of Life*, 2nd ed. New York and Oxford: Oxford University Press.

Blazer, D.G. (2010) 'Protection from late life depression.' *International Psychogeriatrics 22*, 2, 171–173.

Bond, J. and Corner, L. (2006) 'The impact of the label of mild cognitive impairment on the individual's sense of self.' *Philosophy, Psychiatry, & Psychology 13*, 1, 3–12.

Brock, D.W. (1988) 'Justice and the severely demented elderly.' *Journal of Medicine and Philosophy 13*, 1, 73–99.

Clair, A.A. and Memmott, J. (2008) *Therapeutic Uses of Music with Older Adults*, 2nd ed. Silver Spring, MD: American Music Therapy Association.

Coaten, R. (2002) 'Movement matters: Revealing the hidden humanity within dementia through movement, dance and the imagination.' *Dementia: The International Journal of Social Research and Practice 1*, 3, 386–392.

Collerton, J., Davies, K., Jagger, C., Kingston, A. *et al.* (2009) 'Health and disease in 85 year olds: Baseline findings from the Newcastle 85+ cohort study.' *British Medical Journal 399*, b4904.

Dekkers, W.J.M. (2004) 'Autonomy and the Lived Body in Cases of Severe Dementia.' In R.B. Purtilo and H.A.M.J. ten Have (eds) *Ethical Foundations of Palliative Care for Alzheimer Disease*. Baltimore and London: Johns Hopkins University Press.

Dekkers, W. (2010) 'Persons with Severe Dementia and the Notion of Bodily Autonomy.' In J.C. Hughes, M. Lloyd-Williams and G.A. Sachs (eds) *Supportive Care for the Person with Dementia*. Oxford: Oxford University Press.

Department for Constitutional Affairs (2007) *Mental Capacity Act 2005 Code of Practice*. London: The Stationery Office.

Department of Health (n.d.) 'Dementia friendly communities.' *The Dementia Challenge*. Available at http://dementiachallenge.dh.gov.uk/category/areas-for-action/communities/, accessed 6 February 2014.

Dickenson, D. and Fulford, K.W.M. (2000) *In Two Minds: A Casebook of Psychiatric Ethics*. Oxford: Oxford University Press.

Donne, J. (1999) 'Meditation XVII – Nunc Lento Sonitu Dicunt, Morieris.' From *Devotions upon Emergent Occasions and Death's Duel*. New York: Vintage Spiritual Classics. (Original work published 1624.)

Downs, M., Clare, L. and Mackenzie, J. (2006) 'Understandings of Dementia: Explanatory Models and Their Implications for the Person with Dementia and Therapeutic Effort.' In J.C. Hughes, S.J. Louw and S.R. Sabat (eds) *Dementia: Mind, Meaning, and the Person*. Oxford: Oxford University Press.

Emmett, C., Poole, M., Bond, J. and Hughes, J.C. (2013) 'Homeward bound or bound for a home? Assessing the capacity of dementia patients to make decisions about hospital discharge: Comparing practice with legal standards.' *International Journal of Law and Psychiatry 36*, 1, 73–82.

Engel, G.L. (1980) 'The clinical application of the biopsychosocial model.' *American Journal of Psychiatry 137*, 5, 535–544.

Fabiszewski, K.J., Volicer, B. and Volicer, L. (1990) 'Effect of antibiotic treatment on outcome of fevers in institutionalized Alzheimer patients.' *Journal of the American Medical Association 263*, 23, 3168–3172.

Foot, P. (2001) *Natural Goodness*. Oxford: Clarendon Press.

Fratiglioni, L. and Qiu, C. (2013) 'Epidemiology of Dementia.' In T. Dening and A. Thomas (eds) *Oxford Textbook of Old Age Psychiatry*. Oxford: Oxford University Press.

Fulford, K.W.M. (1989) *Moral Theory and Medical Practice*. Cambridge: Cambridge University Press.

Fulford, K.W.M. (2004) 'Facts/Values: Ten Principles of Values-Based Medicine.' In J. Radden (ed.) *The Philosophy of Psychiatry: A Companion*. Oxford: Oxford University Press.

Fulford K.M. and Sayce, L. (1998) 'Invited commentaries on: Mental health legislation is now a harmful anachronism.' *Psychiatric Bulletin 22*, 1, 666–670.

Fulford, K.W.M., Peile, E. and Carroll, H. (2012) *Essentials of Values-Based Practice: Clinical Stories Linking Science with People*. Cambridge: Cambridge University Press.

Fulford, K.W.M., Thornton, T. and Graham, G. (eds) (2006) *Oxford Textbook of Philosophy and Psychiatry*. Oxford: Oxford University Press.

Gombrich, E.H. and Gormley, A.E.H. (2000) 'Gombrich in Conversation with Antony Gormley.' In J. Hutchinson, E.H. Gombrich, L.B. Njatin and W.J.T. Mitchell (eds) *Antony Gormley*, 2nd ed. London: Phaidon Press.

Graham, P. and Hughes J.C. (2014) 'Assisted dying – The debate: *Videtur…sed contra.*' *Advances in Psychiatric Treatment 20*, 4, 250–257.

Gray, D., Proctor, C. and Kirkwood, T. (2013) 'Biological Aspects of Ageing.' In T. Dening and A. Thomas (eds) *Oxford Textbook of Old Age Psychiatry*. Oxford: Oxford University Press.

Greenblat, C. (2012) *Love, Loss, and Laughter: Seeing Alzheimer's Differently*. Guildford, CT: Lyons Press.

Harré, R. (1983) *Personal Being. A Theory for Individual Psychology*. Oxford: Basil Blackwell.

Harris, J. (2005) 'Scientific research is a moral duty.' *Journal of Medical Ethics 31*, 4, 242–248.

Hayes, J. and Povey, S. (2011) *The Creative Arts in Dementia Care: Practical Person-Centred Approaches and Ideas*. London and Philadelphia: Jessica Kingsley Publishers.

Heidegger, M. (1962) *Being and Time* (trans. J. Macquarrie and E. Robinson). Malden, MA, Oxford, and Carlton (Australia): Blackwell. (Original work published 1927 as *Sein und Zeit*.)

Hertogh, C. (2010) 'Advance Care Planning and Palliative Care in Dementia: A View from the Netherlands.' In J.C. Hughes, M. Lloyd-Williams and G.A. Sachs (eds) *Supportive Care for the Person with Dementia*. Oxford: Oxford University Press.

Hodges, J.R. (2007) *Cognitive Assessment for Clinicians*, 2nd ed. Oxford: Oxford University Press.

House of Lords: Select Committee on the Mental Capacity Act 2005 (2014) *Mental Capacity Act 2005: Post-legislative Scrutiny. HL Paper 139*. London: The Stationery Office. Available at www.parliament.uk/mental-capacity-act-2005/, accessed on 14 May 2014.

Hughes, J.C. (2001a) 'Research on Ageing: Implications for Healthcare.' Newcastle Symposium on the Goals of Ageing Research, 24–25 April. Available at www.ncl.ac.uk/peals/assets/symposia/ageing%202001/index.htm, accessed 3 February 2014.

Hughes, J.C. (2001b) 'Views of the person with dementia.' *Journal of Medical Ethics 27*, 2, 86–91.

Hughes, J.C. (ed.) (2005) *Palliative Care in Severe Dementia*. London: Quay Books.

Hughes, J.C. (2006a) 'The heat of mild cognitive impairment.' *Philosophy, Psychiatry, & Psychology 13*, 1, 1–2.

Hughes, J.C. (2006b) 'Patterns of practice: A useful notion in medical ethics?' *Journal of Ethics in Mental Health 1*, 1, 1–5.

Hughes, J.C. (2006c) 'Beyond hypercognitivism: a philosophical basis for good quality palliative care in dementia.' *Supporting and Caring for People with Dementia Throughout End of Life. Les Cahiers de la Fondation Médéric Alzheimer* (June), 17–23.

Hughes, J.C. (2008) 'Searching for settled practice'. *Elderly Client Advise 14*, 1, 26–29.

Hughes, J.C. (2011a) *Thinking Through Dementia*. Oxford: Oxford University Press.

Hughes, J.C. (2011b) *Alzheimer's and Other Dementias: The Facts*. Oxford: Oxford University Press.

Hughes, J.C. (2013a) 'Dementia is Dead, Long Live Ageing: Philosophy and Practice in Connection with "Dementia".' In K.W.M. Fulford, M. Davies, R.G.T. Gipps, G. Graham *et al.* (eds) *Oxford Handbook of Philosophy and Psychiatry*. Oxford: Oxford University Press.

Hughes, J.C. (2013b) 'Paper 35: Models of Dementia Care: Person-Centred, Palliative and Supportive: A Discussion Paper for Alzheimer's Australia on Death and Dying.' *Alzheimer's Australia*. Available at www.fightdementia.org.au/common/files/NAT/Paper_35_web_v2.pdf, accessed 6 February 2014.

Hughes, J.C. and Baldwin, C. (2006) *Ethical Issues in Dementia Care: Making Difficult Decisions*. London and Philadelphia: Jessica Kingsley Publishers.

Hughes, J.C. and Heginbotham, C. (2013) 'Mental Capacity and Decision-Making.' In T. Dening and A. Thomas (eds) *Oxford Textbook of Old Age Psychiatry*. Oxford: Oxford University Press.

Hughes, J.C. and McCormick, A. (2003) 'When to forget is to remember.' *Journal of Dementia Care 11*, 3, 12.

Hughes, J.C., Lloyd-Williams, M., and Sachs, G.A. (eds) (2010) *Supportive Care for the Person with Dementia*. Oxford: Oxford University Press.

Hughes, J.C., Louw, S.J., Sabat, S.R. (2006) 'Seeing Whole.' In J.C. Hughes, S.J. Louw and S.R. Sabat (eds) *Dementia: Mind, Meaning, and the Person*. Oxford: Oxford University Press.

Hughes, J.C., Robinson, L. and Volicer, L. (2005) 'Specialist palliative care in dementia.' *British Medical Journal 330*, 7482, 57–58.

Hughes, J.C., Hope, T., Reader, S. and Rice, D. (2002) 'Dementia and ethics: The views of informal carers.' *Journal of the Royal Society of Medicine 95*, 5, 242–246.

Hughes, J.C., Jolley, D., Jordan, A. and Sampson, E.L. (2007) 'Palliative care in dementia: Issues and evidence.' *Advances in Psychiatric Treatment 13*, 4, 251–260.

Hursthouse, R. (1999) *On Virtue Ethics*. Oxford: Oxford University Press.

Husebo, B.S., Ballard, C., Sandvik, R., Nilsen, O.B. and Aarsland, D. (2011) 'Efficacy of treating pain to reduce behavioural disturbances in residents of nursing homes with dementia: cluster randomised clinical trial.' *British Medical Journal 343*, d4065.

Hutchinson J. (2000) 'Return (The Turning Point).' In J. Hutchinson, E.H. Gombrich, L.B. Njatin and W.J.T. Mitchell (eds) *Antony Gormley*, 2nd ed. London: Phaidon Press.

Ignatieff, M. (2001) *The Needs of Strangers*. New York: Picador. (Original work published 1984.)

Jordan, A.I., Regnard, C. and Hughes, J.C. (2007) 'Hidden pain or hidden evidence?' *Journal of Pain and Symptom Management 33*, 6, 658–660.

Jordan, A., Regnard, C., O'Brien, J.T. and Hughes, J.C. (2012) 'Pain and distress in advanced dementia: Choosing the right tools for the job.' *Palliative Medicine 26*, 7, 873–878.

Jordan, A., Hughes, J., Pakresi, M., Hepburn, S. and O'Brien, J.T. (2011) 'The utility of PAINAD in assessing pain in a UK population with severe dementia.' *International Journal of Geriatric Psychiatry 26*, 2, 118–126.

Keats, J. (1990) *The Major Works* (ed. E. Cook). Oxford: Oxford University Press.

Kennedy, I. (1997) 'Consent: Adult, refusal of consent, capacity. Commentary on Re MB [1997] 2 F.L.R. 426.' *Medical Law Review 5*, 3, 317–325.

Keown, J. (ed.) (1995) *Euthanasia Examined: Ethical, Clinical and Legal Perspectives.* Cambridge: Cambridge University Press.

Killick, J. (2011) 'Becoming a Friend of Time.' In A. Jewell (ed.) *Spirituality and Personhood in Dementia.* London and Philadelphia: Jessica Kingsley Publishers.

Killick, J. (2013a) *Playfulness and Dementia: A Practice Guide.* London and Philadelphia: Jessica Kingsley Publishers.

Killick, J. (2013b) *Dementia Positive: A Handbook Based on Lived Experiences.* Edinburgh: Luath Press.

Killick, J. and Allan K. (2001) *Communication and the Care of People with Dementia.* Buckingham: Open University Press.

Killick, J. and Cordonnier, C. (2000) *Openings: Dementia Poems & Photographs.* London: Journal of Dementia Care and Hawker Publications.

Killick, J. and Craig, C. (2012) *Creativity and Communication in Persons with Dementia: A Practical Guide.* London and Philadelphia: Jessica Kingsley Publishers.

King, Jr, M.L. (1967) 'Speech on receiving his Honorary Doctorate of Civil Law from Newcastle University on 13 November 1967.' *Newcastle University.* Available at www. ncl.ac.uk/congregations/assets/documents/MLKspeech.pdf, accessed 5 February 2014.

Kirkwood, T.B. (2008) 'A systematic look at an old problem.' *Nature 451*, 7179, 644–647.

Kitwood, T. (1997) *Dementia Reconsidered: The Person Comes First.* Buckingham and Philadelphia: Open University Press.

Kontos, P.C. (2006) 'Embodied selfhood. An ethnographic exploration of Alzheimer's disease.' In A. Leibing and L. Cohen (eds) *Thinking About Dementia: Culture, Loss, and the Anthropology of Senility.* Piscataway, New Jersey: Rutgers University Press.

Kontos, P.C. (2004) 'Ethnographic reflections on selfhood, embodiment and Alzheimer's disease.' *Ageing and Society 24*, 6, 829–849.

Lesser, A.H. (2006) 'Dementia and Personal Identity.' In J.C. Hughes, S.J. Louw and S.R. Sabat (eds) *Dementia: Mind, Meaning, and the Person.* Oxford: Oxford University Press.

Locke, J. (1964) *An Essay Concerning Human Understanding* (ed. A.D. Woozley). Glasgow: William Collins/Fount. (Original work published 1690.)

Lord Chancellor's Department (2003) *Making Decisions. Helping People Who Have Difficulty Deciding for Themselves.* London: Lord Chancellor's Department.

Lord Walton of Detchant (1994) *Medical Ethics: Select Committee Report.* House of Lords: *Hansard* 9 May: vol. 554, cc1344–412.

Louw, S.J. and Hughes, J.C. (2005) 'Moral reasoning – the unrealized place of casuistry in medical ethics.' *International Psychogeriatrics 17*, 2 149–154.

Luntley, M. (2002) 'Knowing how to manage: Expertise and embedded knowledge.' *Reasons in Practice 2*, 3, 3–14.

Macquarrie, J. (1968) *Martin Heidegger.* London: Lutterworth Press.

Macquarrie, J. (1972) *Existentialism.* Harmondsworth: Penguin Books.

Matthews, E. (1996) *Twentieth-Century French Philosophy*. Oxford: Oxford University Press.

Matthews, E. (2002) *The Philosophy of Merleau-Ponty*. Chesham: Acumen Publishing.

Matthews, E. (2005) *Mind: Key Concepts in Philosophy*. London and New York: Continuum.

Matthews, E. (2006) 'Dementia and the Identity of the Person.' In J.C. Hughes, S.J. Louw and S.R. Sabat (eds) *Dementia: Mind, Meaning, and the Person*. Oxford: Oxford University Press.

Matthews, E. (2007) *Body-Subjects and Disordered Minds: Treating the Whole Person in Psychiatry*. Oxford: Oxford University Press.

McCulloch, G. (2003) *The Life of the Mind: An Essay on Phenomenological Externalism*. London and New York: Routledge.

McGinn, C. (1989) *Mental Content*. Oxford: Blackwell.

McMillan, J. (2006) 'Identity, Self and Dementia.' In J.C. Hughes, S.J. Louw and S.R. Sabat (eds) *Dementia: Mind, Meaning, and the Person*. Oxford: Oxford University Press.

Merleau-Ponty, M. (1962) *Phenomenology of Perception* (trans. C. Smith). London and New York: Routledge. (Original work published as *Phénomènologie de la Perception* in 1945.)

Midgley, M. (2001) *Science and Poetry*. London and New York: Routledge.

Ministry of Justice (2008) *Mental Capacity Act 2005 Deprivation of Liberty Safeguards: Code of Practice to Supplement the Main Mental Capacity Act 2005 Code of Practice*. London: The Stationery Office.

Mitchell, S.L., Teno, J.M., Kiely, D.K., Shaffer, M.L. *et al.* (2009) 'The clinical course of advanced dementia.' *New England Journal of Medicine 361*, 16, 1529–1538.

Moreira, T., Hughes, J.C., Kirkwood, T., May, C., McKeith, I. and Bond, J. (2008) 'What explains variations in the clinical use of mild cognitive impairment (MCI) as a diagnostic category?' *International Psychogeriatrics 20*, 4, 697–709.

Nuffield Council on Bioethics (2009) *Dementia: Ethical Issues*. London: Nuffield Council on Bioethics.

O'Brien, J.T. and Grayson, L. (2013) 'Mild Cognitive Impairment and Predementia Syndromes.' In T. Dening and A. Thomas (eds) *Oxford Textbook of Old Age Psychiatry*, 2nd ed. Oxford: Oxford University Press.

Oppenheimer, C. (2006) 'I Am, Thou Art: Personal Identity in Dementia.' In J.C. Hughes, S.J. Louw and S.R. Sabat (eds) *Dementia: Mind, Meaning, and the Person*. Oxford: Oxford University Press.

Ottaway, S.R. (2004) *The Decline of Life: Old Age in Eighteenth-Century England*. Cambridge: Cambridge University Press.

Parfit, D. (1984) *Reasons and Persons*. Oxford: Oxford University Press.

Percy Commission (1957) *Report of the Royal Commission on the Law Relating to Mental Illness and Mental Deficiency 1954–1957 (Cmnd 169)*. London: HMSO.

Pointon, B. (2007) 'Who am I? – The Search for Spirituality in Dementia: A Family Carer's Perspective.' In M.E. Coyte, P. Gilbert and V. Nicholls (eds) *Spirituality, Values and Mental Health: Jewels for the Journey*. London and Philadelphia: Jessica Kingsley Publishers.

Polanyi, M. (1958) *Personal Knowledge: Towards a Post-Critical Philosophy*. London: Routledge & Kegan Paul.

Post, S.G. (1995) *The Moral Challenge of Alzheimer Disease.* Baltimore and London: Johns Hopkins University Press.

Post, S.G. (2000) *The Moral Challenge of Alzheimer Disease: Ethical Issues from Diagnosis to Dying,* 2nd ed. Baltimore and London: Johns Hopkins University Press.

Post, S.G. (2006) 'Respectare: Moral Respect for the Lives of the Deeply Forgetful.' In J.C. Hughes, S.J. Louw and S.R. Sabat (eds) *Dementia: Mind, Meaning, and the Person.* Oxford: Oxford University Press.

Regnard, C., Reynolds, J., Watson, B., Matthews, D., Gibson, L. and Clarke C. (2007) 'Understanding distress in people with severe communication difficulties: Developing and assessing the disability distress assessment tool DisDAT.' *Journal of Intellectual Disability Research 51,* 4, 277–292. DisDAT is available at http://disdattool.wordpress.com, accessed 6 February 2014.

Richards, M. and Brayne, C. (2010) 'What do we mean by Alzheimer's disease?' *British Medical Journal 341,* 4670, 865–867.

Robinson, L., Dickinson, C., Bamford, C., Clark, A., Hughes, J. and Exley, C. (2013) 'A qualitative study: professionals' experiences of advance care planning in dementia and palliative care, *"a good idea in theory but…".' Palliative Medicine 27,* 5, 401–408.

Sabat, S.R. (2001) *The Experience of Alzheimer's Disease: Life through a Tangled Veil.* Oxford: Blackwell.

Sabat, S.R. (2006) 'Mind, Meaning, and Personhood in Dementia: The Effects of Positioning.' In J.C. Hughes, S.J. Louw and S.R. Sabat (eds) *Dementia: Mind, Meaning, and the Person.* Oxford: Oxford University Press.

Sabat, S.R. and Harré, R. (1994) 'The Alzheimer's disease sufferer as a semiotic subject.' *Philosophy, Psychiatry, & Psychology 1,* 3, 145–160.

Sadler, J.Z. (2004) *Values and Psychiatric Diagnosis.* Oxford: Oxford University Press.

Sampson, E.L., Gould, V., Lee, D. and Blanchard, M.R. (2006) 'Differences in care received by patients with and without dementia who died during acute hospital admission: A retrospective case note study.' *Age & Ageing 35,* 1, 187–189.

Sampson, E.L., Blanchard, M.R., Jones, L., Tookman, A. and King, M. (2009) 'Dementia in the acute hospital: Prospective cohort study of prevalence and mortality.' *British Journal of Psychiatry 195,* 2, 61–66.

Shega, J.W. and Sachs, G.A. (2010) 'Offering Supportive Care in Dementia: Reflections on the PEACE Programme.' In J.C. Hughes, M. Lloyd-Williams and G.A. Sachs (eds) *Supportive Care for the Person with Dementia.* Oxford: Oxford University Press.

Shega, J.W., Levin, A., Hougham, G.W., Cox-Hayley, D. *et al.* (2003) 'Palliative excellence in Alzheimer care efforts (PEACE): A program description.' *Journal of Palliative Medicine 6,* 315–320.

Snowdon, D.A. (2003) 'Healthy aging and dementia: Findings from the Nun Study.' *Annals of Internal Medicine 139,* 450–454.

Snyder, L. (2006) 'Personhood and Interpersonal Communication in Dementia.' In J.C. Hughes, S.J. Louw and S.R. Sabat (eds) *Dementia: Mind, Meaning, and the Person.* Oxford: Oxford University Press.

Szmukler, G. and Holloway, F. (1998) 'Mental health legislation is now a harmful anachronism.' *Psychiatric Bulletin 22,* 11, 662–665.

Taylor, C. (1989) *Sources of the Self: The Making of the Modern Identity.* Cambridge: Cambridge University Press.

Taylor, C. (1991) *The Ethics of Authenticity.* Cambridge, MA: Harvard University Press.

Taylor, C. (1995) *Philosophical arguments*. Cambridge, MA: Harvard University Press.

Thornton, T. (2006) 'The Discursive Turn, Social Constructionism and Dementia.' In J.C. Hughes, S.J. Louw and S.R. Sabat (eds) *Dementia: Mind, Meaning, and the Person*. Oxford: Oxford University Press.

Thornton, T. (2007) *Essential Philosophy of Psychiatry*. Oxford: Oxford University Press.

Thornton, T. (2013) 'Clinical Judgment, Tacit Knowledge, and Recognition in Psychiatric Diagnosis.' In K.W.M. Fulford, M. Davies, R.G.T. Gipps, G. Graham, G. Stamghellini and T. Thornton (eds) *The Oxford Handbook of Philosophy and Psychiatry*. Oxford: Oxford University Press.

Treloar, A. and Crugel, M. (2010) 'Living and Dying at Home with Dementia.' In J.C. Hughes, M. Lloyd-Williams and G.A. Sachs (eds) *Supportive Care for the Person with Dementia*. Oxford: Oxford University Press.

van der Steen, J. (2010) 'Dying with dementia: What we know after more than a decade of research.' *Journal of Alzheimer's Disease 22*, 1, 37–55.

van der Steen, J.T., Ooms, M.E., Van der Wal, G., Ribbe, M. W. (2002a) 'Pneumonia: The demented patient's best friend? Discomfort after starting or withholding antibiotic treatment.' *Journal of American Geriatrics Society 50*, 10, 1681–1688.

van der Steen, J.T., Ooms, M.E., Mehr, D.R., van der Wal, G. *et al.* (2002b) 'Severe dementia and adverse outcomes of nursing home-acquired pneumonia: Evidence for mediation by functional and pathophysiological decline.' *Journal of the American Geriatrics Society 50*, 439–448.

van der Steen, J.T., Radbruch, L., Hertogh, C.M., de Boer, M.E. *et al.* on behalf of the European Association for Palliative Care (EAPC) (2013) 'White paper defining optimal palliative care in older people with dementia: A Delphi study and recommendations from the European Association for Palliative Care.' *Palliative Medicine*, November.

Vellinga, A., Smit, J.H., van Leeuwen, E., van Tillburg, W. and Jonker, C. (2004) 'Instruments to assess decision-making capacity: An overview.' *International Psychogeriatrics 16*, 4, 397–419.

Volicer, L. and Hurley, A. (1998) *Hospice Care for Patients with Advanced Progressive Dementia*. New York: Springer.

Welsh, S.F. and Keeling, A. (2013) 'The Deprivation of Liberty Safeguards.' In R. Jacob, M. Gunn and A. Holland (eds) *Mental Capacity Legislation: Principles and Practice*. London: RCPsych Publications.

Whitehouse, P.J. and George, D. (2008) *The Myth of Alzheimer's: What You Aren't Being Told about Today's Most Dreaded Diagnosis*. New York: St Martin's Press.

Widdershoven, G.A.M. and Berghmans, R.L.P. (2006) 'Meaning-Making in Dementia: A Hermeneutic Perspective.' In J.C. Hughes, S.J. Louw and S.R. Sabat (eds) *Dementia: Mind, Meaning, and the Person*. Oxford: Oxford University Press.

Williams, B. (1973) *Problems of the Self*. Cambridge: Cambridge University Press.

Wittgenstein, L. (1958) *The Blue and Brown Books*. Oxford: Blackwell.

Wittgenstein, L. (1968) *Philosophical Investigations* (ed. G.E.M Anscombe and R. Rhees, trans. G.E.M. Anscombe). Oxford: Blackwell.

Wittgenstein, L. (1969) *On Certainty* (ed. G.E.M. Anscombe and G.H. von Wright, trans. D. Paul and G.E.M. Anscombe). Oxford: Blackwell.

Wittgenstein, L. (1980) *Culture and Value* (ed. G.H. von Wright and H. Nyman, trans. P. Winch). Oxford: Blackwell.

Wittgenstein, L. (1992) *Last Writings on the Philosophy of Psychology. Volume II. The Inner and The Outer, 1949–1951* (ed. G.H. von Wright and H. Nyman, trans. C.G. Luckhardt and M.A.E. Aue). Oxford: Blackwell.

Wordsworth, W. (2000) *The Major Works* (ed. S. Gill). Oxford: Oxford University Press.

Zeisel, J. (2009) *I'm Still Here: A New Philosophy of Alzheimer's Care.* New York: Avery.

Zwakhalen, S.M., van der Steen, J. and Najim, M.D. (2012) 'Which score most likely represents pain on the observational PAINAD pain scale for patients with dementia?' *Journal of the American Medical Directors Association 13*, 4, 384–389.

Legal References

B v Croydon Health Authority [1995] Fam 133

CoA [2011] EWCA Civ 190

HL v United Kingdom (2004) 40 EHRR 761

JE v DE and Surrey County Council (2006) EWHC 3459 (Fam)

P (by his litigation friend the Official Solicitor) (Appellant) v Cheshire West and Chester Council and another (Respondents); P and Q (by their litigation friend, the Official Solicitor) (Appellants) v Surrey County Council (Respondent) [2014] UKSC 19 On appeal from [2011] EWCA Civ 1257; [2011] EWCA Civ 190

R v Bournewood Community and Mental Health NHS Trust, ex parte L [1998] 3 AllER 289

Further Reading

On ageing

Kirkwood, T. (1999) *Time of Our Lives: The Science of Human Ageing*. London: Phoenix.

Small, H. (2007) *The Long Life*. Oxford: Oxford University Press.

On personhood

Gillett, G. (2008) *Subjectivity and Being Someone: Human Identity and Neuroethics*. Exeter: Imprint Academic.

Capacity and incapacity

Watt, H. (ed.) (2009) *Incapacity and Care: Controversies in Healthcare and Research*. Oxford: Linacre Centre.

Palliative and supportive care

Small, N., Froggatt, K. and Downs, M. (2008) *Living and Dying with Dementia: Dialogues about Palliative Care*. Oxford: Oxford University Press.

The arts

Sacks, O. (2007) *Musicophilia: Tales of Music and the Brain*. London: Picador.

Storr, A. (1992) *Music and the Mind*. New York: Free Press.

Subject Index

Page numbers referring to footnotes are followed by *n*. Page numbers for Figures or Boxes are shown in *italics*.

acquired diffuse neurocognitive dysfunction 11
action
    embodied 227
    intention embodied/inherent in 195–6
    intentional 195
    involves intentional nature 187, 195
    nature of 196
    pursues a purpose 195–6
Adults with Incapacity (Scotland) Act 72
advance care planning 46–7, 118–19, 167, 182
    see also Mental Capacity Act
Advance Decisions to Refuse Treatment *see*
    Mental Capacity Act
advance directives 193
aesthetic
    appreciation 21
    approach 225
    reaction to the world 220
    response 23
    sense 228
    understanding of personhood 143, 145
ageing 18
    and dementia 39–42
    normal 39–42
    research 35, 36–9, 41, 54
    paradigm 42
    possibilities 226
    problematic 226
age-related diseases 36
agency
    situated 190
Alzheimer's 11, 39–40, 43, 50, 58, 60, 166, 206, 216
    senile plaques 206
    Society 48 *see also* dementia
antibiotics 168, 169
anti-dementia drugs 190
antidepressant *113*
art 23
    and dementia 23, 202
    commemoration 209

creative relationships 204
    encourages broad view 202
    practice involves give and take 203–4
Art Mama 216
artificial nutrition and hydration 169
Arts and Humanities Research Council 13
Arts Council of England 15
assessment
    clinical 103–106
assisted dying 183–4
atavism 52–4
atomism 132, 137, 213
attentional skills 163–4
autonomy 78, 106, 128
    bodily 86, 89
    dependence 123–4
    interests *67*
    importance of 105
    Lasting Powers of Attorney (LPA) 117
    professional 118
    rational 87
    respect for 117
    well-being and 48, 67

Beamish Museum 60–61
beauty 220
being
    aesthetic 221
    as human beings 34, 225
    in the moment 223
    -in-the-world 22, 65, 77, 139, 227, 228
    of this kind/type 33
    moment-to-moment 32
    situated embodied agent and 214
    -with-others 64, 77, 139
    -with-the-other-in-the-moment 225
    with/doing to 143, 228
beliefs 68, 138
    background 139
    competence and 95
    personal 138
    religious 138, 171
    scientific 161
best interests 17, 18, 43, 99, 105, *110–11*, *113*, 115, *116*, 128, 186, 189, 198

absence of capacity 106
broad view 192–3
deprivation of liberty 123
Independent Mental Capacity Advocate
    (IMCA) 119–20
palliative care and 187
pausing 115
restraint 121
the SEA view and 192–4,
see also Mental Capacity Act
body 20, 34, 71, 76–90, 161, 187, 188
articulates meaning 214
general medium for having a world 76, 79,
    80, 89, 213, 214
language 152
lived 86–8
politic 21
significance of 78
-subject 77–80, 81, 83, 103, 148
understands 79–80
see also embodiment; Merleau-Ponty; person
borderline personality disorder 131
boundedness
see life
Bournewood
gap 133
Hospital 120
Breadmen 215

Camera Lucida 211
see also Barthes, R.
capacity 113, 131
approaches to assessment of capacity 93–5
assessment as externalist 106
cognitive 95, 104, 106, 108
complexity 128
definition 92, 99, 100, 101
human rights 99
legalistic view 20
legal tests 104
metaphysical question 99
residence 92, 99
tests 104
values 92
see also competence; decision-making;
    incapacity; Mental Capacity Act
cardiopulmonary resuscitation 169
care 18, 32
concrete manifestations of
for human being 18
health and social 51
in world with others 227
homes 51
long-term 104
models of 18
new culture of dementia 221
pathway 183
pathway (Liverpool) 180
person-centred 18, 176, 178, 189

political 228
priorities at the end of life 177
psychosocial aspects 19
supportive care 179, 182
see also palliative
carers
family 197
natural reactions 197
case examples
Mr Adams 96–7
Mr Bowes 68–9, 71, 73–4, 76, 77, 86, 87
Mrs George 110–11, 112
Mr Jenkins 113, 114–5, 116
Mrs Krasinska 116, 117
Mrs Sengupta 130–1, 139
casuistry 171–2
causal accounts 34 see also consciousness;
    memory
citizens 21, 65
clinician
pulled to community 204
coherence
internal 171
external 171–2
collective
subjective 214
unconscious 145
commitment
individual 229
political 229
communication 61, 176, 216
and relationships 21
authentic 225
deep 223
end of life 193
community 53–4
dementia-friendly 75
endeavour 229
living in the 104
competence
evaluative 95, 104
volitional 95, 104
see also capacity
complexity 21, 133, 136
concept 209–13
concern 215–7
connoisseurship 160–1, 164
consciousness 21, 56–7
causal account 56–7
constitutive account 56–7
human 21, 142, 144–6
self- 21, 142, 144, 145–6
consent 106, 128, 129, 132
capacity to consent 43
constitutive accounts 34
see also consciousness; memory
content 213–5
context 205–9, 221

covert medication *113*
creative arts 217

dance 217
decision-making 43, 95, 96, 97, 104–8, 112,
     115, *116*, 118, 124
   capacity 13, 20, 72, 92, 94
   ethical 170
   personhood 72
   proxy 47
   shared 118, 174, *175*, *176*
   values 20
   volitional nature 104
   whole person 20
   see also capacity; Mental Capacity Act
Dasein 102
death
   as natural part of life 193
defectology 189, 208–9
   see also Sabat, S.
dementia 130, 134
   and ageing 19, 39–42
   cannot morally disregard people with 187,
      198
   concept 23
   definition 11–12
   early diagnosis 46–8, 51
   friendly communities 43
   harmful *67*
   how we think about it 10
   moral standing of people with 143
   part of ageing 45
   quality of life *67*
   research 35, 42, 54
   severe 15, 33, 47, 60, 70–2, 76, 78, 81,
      86–7, 88–90, 142, 143, 149–50, 151,
      152–3, 158, 164, 168–70, 171, 184,
      186, 188, 189, 190–1, 197–8, 213,
      215
   stigmatizing 42
   syndrome 42
   terminal condition 166
   timely diagnosis 48
   vascular *96 see also* ageing; Alzheimer's
dependence
   and autonomy 123–4
depression 31–2
deprivation of liberty 18, 120–4, 135
   imputable to the state 123
   normality 123
   objective and subjective elements 123
   safeguards (DoLS) 120–1, 124, 125, 126*n see
      also* best interests
diabetes *110*, 111
Diagnostic and Statistical Manual (DSM-5) 11,
      49, 136
DisDAT 153–5, 164
distress 48, 112, 131, 153–9, 161–4, 166, 168,
      219

language of 157–9, 161, 164
dorsolateral prefrontal cortex 59
dorsolateral striatum 58
dotage 19, 54
double effect 194

eating problems *166*
economics 19
embodied
   selfhood 84–5, 89, 221
   subjectivities 227
embodiment 83, 84, 196, 214 *see also* body
emotional response 23
emotions 21
end of life 14, 18, 20, 22, 149, 165, 170, 193–4
Endymion 219
Essential Philosophy of Psychiatry 156
esthetic *see* aesthetic
ethical
   case-based decisions *67*
   framework *67*, 71
   imperative 46, 52
   see also Ordinary and Extraordinary Means;
      research; treatment; values; virtues
European Association for Palliative Care 173
European Convention on Human Rights 120
European Court 120–1, 122
euthanasia 183–4, 186, 191, 197
Externalism *see* mind

facial expression 152, 155
false positives 153–4
fever *166*
flourishing 38, 43, 172–3, 183–4, 222
Fondation Médéric Alzheimer 6
force-feeding 131–2
forgetfulness
   pathological depends on the social context
      207
   not in itself pathological, depending on
      consequences and context 206
form(s) of life 28, 159
functional illness 134

gaze 220
gestures 72, 190 *see* meaning
Glimpses 222
Gross Domestic Profit 50

habit 79–80
habitus 84
hippocampus 58
historical view 52
holism
   and SEA view 193
hypercognitivism 71, 142–3, 148, 150, 221

incapacity 21, *100*, 128
Independent Mental Capacity Advocate
    (IMCA) *see* best interests; Mental
    Capacity Act
intentionality *see* mind
Intention 195
intentions 194
    and foreseen consequences 194
    not inner 186, 198
interaction
    and concern 217
interconnectedness 23, 202, 224, 216, 217, 223
inter-dependence 32
interpretation 63, 107–8, 147, 156–8, 161,
    162, 191, 227 *see also* judgement
inter–relate 64, 188, 202
inter-relationship 124
intuition 11, 100, 138, 155, 139, 220, 222
Iraq war 224
I-Thou relationships *see* Buber
"It's a long way to Tipperary" 215

Joan
    meaningful activity 215
Journal of Mental Health Law 129
joy 219
judgement 11, 105, 106, 112, 177, 191
    about decision-making 20–1, 95–6, 106,
        107, 129, 131
    about intentions 23
    background of complex interrelationships
        138
    clinical 22, 48, 110, 111, 118–9, 139, 152,
        158, 162–3, 164, 168, 184
    emotional 95
    ethical 35
    global, about capacities 111
    legal 120, 121, 122, 123, 126*n*, 133, 134,
        137
    of an action 187, 198
    professional 109, 115, 117, 138
    tacit component of 155–9
    within language 161
    value 40–1, 95, 104, 107, 108, 131

language 226
Lasting Powers of Attorney *see* Mental Capacity
    Act
law *101*, 106–8, 139
legal cases
    B v Croydon Health Authority [1995] Fam
        133 131
    CoA [2011] EWCA Civ 190 122
    HL v United Kingdom (2004) 40 EHRR 761
        121–2
    JE v and DE Surrey County Council 121
    *P v Cheshire West and Chester Council and
        another; P and Q v Surrey County
        Council* [2014] UKSC 19 126*n*

*R v Bournewood Community and Mental
    Health NHS Trust*, exparte L [1998]
    3 AllER 289 133
letting go 197
life
    as a good 187, 197
    bounded 28, 31, 51
    narrative 31
    quality 36–7, 38
    quantity 36, 38
limit situation 30
living wills 193
longevity 27
Lord Chancellor's Department 97
lost property
    glasses 210, 212

Making Decisions Alliance 127
malignant positioning 178 *see also* Sabat, S.
malignant social psychology 178, 189 *see also*
    Kitwood, T.
Man Friday 102
meaning
    as use 28
    contextual 72
    conveying 222
    in extreme frailty 33
    in public space 63
    gestures 72, 75, 190
    through our bodies 79
    see also significance
meaningful activities 61
memory 64
    and person 69–70
    and forgetting 212
    anterograde 58
    causal account 57–61
    constitutive account 61
    emotional 59, 145
    episodic 58, 144
    essentially shareable 213
    implicit 145
    loss 19, 56–65
    phenomenological experience 61
    potentially shareable 63
    procedural 58
    retrograde 58
    semantic 58, 59
    understanding 56
    working 59
MEG 122–3, 126*n*
memorials 209
Mental Capacity Act 2005 (MCA) 12, 72, 93,
    96, 109–26
    advance care planning 119
    Advance Decisions to Refuse Treatment 118
    ageing 18
    best interests *116*, 128, 193
    Code of Practice 114

Mental Capacity Act 2005 (MCA) *cont.*
  complexity 111–12
  definition of lack of capacity 99, *100*
  distinction between MCA and MHA 127–8,
      130–1, 139
  House of Lords Select Committee 126*n*
  Independent Mental Capacity Advocate
      (IMCA) 119
  Lasting Powers of Attorney 47, 117, 128
  problems of implementation 115, 126*n*
  restraint 120–1
  section 2(1) *100*
  section 3(1) *100*
  sections 5 and 6 120
  tension in 109
  unwarranted interference in practice 110
mental disorder 21, 82, 98, 127–139
  as a subset of mental incapacity 135
  mental incapacity as subset of 134 *see also*
      Mental Health Act
Mental Health Act 1983 (MHA) 54, 98, 120,
      127–36, 139
  broad definition of mental disorder 128
  compulsory treatment 130
  medical treatment 132
  section 3 131
  sections 57 and 58 132
  section 63 132
  section 131(1) 134
  section 145(1) 132
mental life
  goes on in external space 147
  socially embedded 188
Metropolitan Opera, New York 27
MIG 122–3, 126*n*
Mild Cognitive Impairment (MCI) 49, 208
mind
  being minded 148
  constitutive feature 63
  external 19, 22, 61, 63, 77, 142, 146–7, 148,
      149–50, 170, 213
  inner 213
  intentionality of 61, 146
  outer processes 213
  social constructionists 77
Mind: Key Concepts in Philosophy 77
models 178–9
  biopsychosocial 178
  spiritual and biopsychosocial 178–9
  see also care; palliative; world
morbidity curve
  rectangularization 37
Mr B 209
museum 60–1, 64, 217
music 20, 30, 59, 64, 79–80, 143, 145, 217,
      222, 227
Mystery 222, 225

Nae Oniebody 224
narrative 148, 213
naso-gastric tube 87–8
National Dementia Strategy for England 51
negative capability 219, 221, 222
negative vocalizations 153, 156
neighbours *96–7*, 103
neuroimaging 58
neuropathology 206
neuropsychologists
  cognitive 58
Newcastle
  consultation on memorials 210
  Earl Grey monument 224
Newcastle University
  85+ Study 38
  Hatton Gallery 14
  'Holding Memories' Workshop 12
  Policy, Ethics and Life Sciences (PEALS)
      Research Institute 12, 14 *see also* King
      Jr, Martin Luther
no ifs, ands, or buts 210, *211*
normative 62, 63, 102, 157, 171
normativity 61, 62–3, 183
  platonic 62–3
  social constructionism 63
Northern Print Studio 14
Nuffield Council on Bioethics 6, 13, 66, 71, 72
  ethical framework *67*, 75
  living well with dementia 17
  timely diagnosis 47–8
Nun study 206
nursing
  need for exceptional skills in dementia 191
Nursing Times 15

occupational therapist *97*
On Certainty 158–9
Ordinary and Extraordinary Means
  Doctrine of 169–70, 177–8
organic disorder 134
Other 220, 222
Oxford Textbook of Philosophy and Psychiatry 159

pain 14, 22, 76, 146, 151–5, 156, 162, 163,
      164, 166, 167, 168, 190, 220
  behaviour 152–3
  management *182*
PAINAD 152–5, 164
painting 221
palliative 17–18, 51
  approach 167, 186–7, 198
  care 14, 18, 46, 86, 142, 143, 150, 151,
      165–8, 173–5, *176*, 178–80, 183, 187,
      191, 193–194, 198–9
  measure 168
  sedation 198
  see also white paper
parentalism 112

paternalism 109, 112
pause 115
people-in-the-world 138
percutaneous endoscopic gastrostomy (PEG) tube 87–8, *116*, 117
Percy Commission 134
person 63, 66–75
 affective 142
 amongst persons 228
 and body 20
 and dementia 22
 as agents 188
 as minded 148
 cannot be circumscribed 187
 decisions for 18
 embedded in the world 196
 identity *67*, 70, 88
 memory 69–70
 relational 142
 situated embodied agent (SEA) 19–20, 63–4, 74, 103, 149, 184, 186, 191, 196, 213, 217, 221, 226
 valued *67*
 with dementia as semiotic subject 189
 personal identity *see* person
personhood 18, 19, 66, *67*, 74, 82, 142, 145
 broad view of 75, 142, 188
 enhancing 150
 maintained by meaningful activity 64
 persists into severe dementia 191, 198
 see also person
Phenomenology of Perception 79, 89
philosophical
 clarity 133, 136–8
 confusion 133–6
Philosophical Investigations 152, 156, 157
Philosophy 13, 17, 63, 70, 77, 101, 164, 167, 205
 analytic 187
 and practice 81, 96, 100
 continental 187
photography
 "a new science for each object" 211
 "impossible science of the unique being" 212
 representation 211
 see also Barthes
physician-assisted suicide 186, 191, 197
play 221
pneumonia *116*, *166*, 168
poetry 221
polis 109, 120, 125, 228
politics 19
post–traumatic stress disorder 131
pottery 221
practical
 know-how 103, 104, 158
 knowledge 101, 103, 105, 160
practice 102

human worldly 63
 patterns of 22, 137, 138, 159, 165, 170–3, 184
 professional 115
pre-understanding 159
Psychiatric Bulletin 128
psychiatrist *97*, 130
psychoanalytic psychotherapy 132
psychology
 cognitive 188
 social 188
psychopathic disorder 132
psychotic 129, 133

research 19
 applied 43
 basic 43
 duty to participate 50
 ethical imperative 46
 participatory action 44
 right to participate 50
 translational 43–45
revolution 64–5, 225
risk 105
Robinson Crusoe 102
Royal College of Psychiatrists 13
rules 102, 157, 160, 163

Sciart
 Consortium 15
 'Memory and Forgetting' 14, 202, 203, 223
science
 reductionist 204
 seeing 203
 simplifying 203
SEA view of person *see* person
sedimentation 84–5, 86, 87
self-harm 131
selfhood
 embodied 85, 89, 221
 see also personhood
significance 20, 22, 28, 33–4, 64, 184
 because of context 27, 29
 gestural 84, 86, 87
 horizon of 184
 human 75, 172
 of body 78
 of final years 18, 27, 30, 31
 of our lives 18, 229
 moral or ethical 227
 person of 54, 81
 personal 209
 political 227
 world has 85
Single Photon Emission Computed Tomography (SPECT) scan 210, 212
situated embodied agents *see* personhood
society
 individualistic 216

sociology 19
Solicitors for the Elderly 6
solicitude 23, 32–3, 34, 65, 75, 90, 212, 215,
    226–9
solidarity 65, *67*, 75, 228–9
solipsism 77
spiritual
    approach 223
    see also models; world
stroke *116*
Supportive Care for the Person with Dementia 86

tacit knowledge 85, 86, 88, 158–62 *see also*
    judgement
tangles
    glasses 210
    neurofibrillary 210
temporal lobe
    anterior 59
The Blue Book 152
The Experience of Alzheimer's Disease 60
The Fountain 229
The Makropulos Affair 26–7, 29
The Two Thieves, or The Last Stage of Avarice
    53–54
Thinking Through Dementia 11, 40
treatment
    withholding and withdrawing 166–70
truth 220

uncertainty *110*, 114–5, 118, 170, 225
urinal 205, 207

value–laden
    acts 92, 102, 103, 105, 107, 108
    diagnoses 134
    questions 130
values 41, 208
    -based practice 180–2,
    diverse 21
    facts and 21, 23
    mental disorder and mental illness 137
    personal 138
    worldly context of 21
virtues 171–2
    define as moral agents 197
vocalization 190

wandering 130
well-being *67 see also* quality of life
white paper on optimal palliative care for older
    people with dementia 173–8
world 20, 22, 28, 33, 44–5, 56, 57, 78, 79,
    102, 107, 124, 127, 148–50, 183–4, 188,
    196, 206, 214–5, 217, 219, 220, 221,
    225, 226–8
    aesthetic view/perception 23, 219
    approach to 220
    art 205
    being persons in 63–4, 66, 68

body 81
    capturing the 205
    dementia as in-the- 219
    enters constitutively into states of mind 146
    external 142, 147, 227
    how we see the 219
    human 22, 34, 75, 82, 92, 102–3, 105,
        107, 108
    human beings in the 10
    in terms of beauty 219
    inner 227
    meaning 34, 54, 79
    mental states peoples by the 62
    moral 74
    of others 75, 207
    of relations 105
    one, but a big one 127, 137, 138
    person 103
    science as simplifying 203
    self in 146
    shapes our understanding 73
    shared 172
    significance 85
    situatedness in 75
    social 74, 77, 82
    spiritual 103
    understanding located in the 204
    understanding of 136
    values 106
    without models 179–80
    see also being; body

Author Index

Agich, G. 112, 123–4
Allan, K. 15, 216
Anscombe, E. 195
Aristotle 30

Baldwin, C. 10, 11
Barthes, R. 202, 211–2
Bavidge, M. 14, 32
Bellhouse, J. 129–30
Blazer, D. 31–2
Bourdieu, P. 84
Brock, D. 69
Buber, M. 81, 189

Cameron, D. 17
Čapek, K. 26

Dekkers, W. 14, 86–8
Descartes, R. 78
Donne, J. 184–5
Duchamp, M. 202, 205, 207

Emmett, C. 13

Filkin, L. 127–8, 131
Fulford, B. 41, 107, 128–9, 130, 135, 136, 137, 159, 180–1

Gadamer, H–G. 159
Gormley, A. 202, 213–4
Gough, L. 134
Graham, P. 186
Greenblat, C. 216
Ground, I. 14

Harré, R. 188
Heginbotham, C. 13
Heidegger, M. 32–3, 34, 64, 73, 77, 82, 102, 202, 212, 215, 216, 227
Hertogh, C. 168–9
Hoffmann, L.J. 132, 137
Holloway, F. 128, 130

Ignatieff, M. 124–5

Jaspers, K. 30
Janáček, L. 26
Jordan, A. 14

Jung, K. 145

Keats, J. 219–21
Keown, J. 186
Killick, J. 6, 15, 216, 221–5
King Jr, M.L. 125–6
Kirkwood, T. 12
Kitwood, T. 71, 81, 144, 178, 189, 221
Kontos, P. 84–6, 87, 221

Lesser, H. 28–9
Locke, J. 69, 82–3, 187
Louw, S. 14, 70, 171
Luntley, M. 162–4

McCormick, A. 6, 14, 202, 217–8
McCulloch, G. 146–7
Makropulos, E. 26, 30
Makropulos, H. 26
Matthews, E. 13, 77, 78, 81–4, 85–7, 88–9
Merleau-Ponty, M. 76, 77, 78–81, 82, 84, 86, 87, 88, 89, 103, 148, 202, 214
Midgley, M. 14, 137, 138–9
Mitchell, S. 166
Munby, J. 121–2

Orimoto, T. 6, 15, 202, 215–6

Parfit, D. 69, 82–3, 187, 202
Plato 30, 125
Pointon, B. 33
Pointon, M. 33
Polanyi, M. 159–64
Post, S. 71, 142–3, 145, 150, 188, 190, 217, 221

Regnard, C. 14
Ribot, T. 60

Sabat, S. 14, 60, 70, 77, 86, 108, 144, 145, 147, 178, 188–9, 208–9, 221
Sachs, G. 167
Sadler, J. 136
Sampson, E. 167–8
Sayce, L. 128–9, 130
Shakespeare, T. 12
Shega, J. 167

Steyn, L. 133, 134
Szmukler, G. 128, 130

Taylor, C. 31, 34, 85, 184, 187
Thornton, T. 85, 156, 158, 159, 207

van der Steen, J. 6, 14, 167, 173
Versalle, R. 27n
Volicer, L. 166, 191

Walton, L. 196
Whitehouse, P. 40
Williams, B. 29–30
Wittgenstein, L. 28, 63, 72, 73, 77, 152, 154,
        156–8, 159, 161, 162, 163, 187, 195,
        202–3, 205, 213, 214–5
Wordsworth, W. 53–4, 229

Zeisel, J. 217